THIRD EDITION

Easy EMG

A Guide to Performing Nerve Conduction Studies and Electromyography

Authors

LYN D. WEISS MD

Chair of Physical Medicine and Rehabilitation
NYU Langone Hospital Long Island
Professor of Rehabilitation Medicine
NYU Long Island School of Medicine
Mineola, NY, USA

JAY M. WEISS MD

Long Island Physical Medicine and
  Rehabilitation
Jericho, NY, USA
Associate Professor of Clinical Physical
  Medicine and Rehabilitation
State University of New York Stony Brook
  College of Medicine
Stony Brook, NY, USA

JULIE K. SILVER MD

Associate Professor
Department of Physical Medicine and
  Rehabilitation
Harvard Medical School
Boston, MA, USA

Illustrator

DENNIS J. DOWLING DO FAAO

Director of Osteopathic Medicine
  Services
Department of Physical Medicine and
  Rehabilitation
Family Medicine Department
Nassau University Medical Center
East Meadow, NY, USA
Director of OMM Assessment
National Board Osteopathic Medical
  Examiners
Conshohocken, PA, USA

For additional online content visit expertconsult

ELSEVIER   London, New York, Oxford, Philadelphia, St Louis, Sydney, Toronto

Elsevier
1600 John F. Kennedy Blvd.
Ste 1800
Philadelphia, PA 19103-2899

EASY EMG, THIRD EDITION

ISBN: 978-0-323-79686-6

Previous editions copyrighted 2016, 2004.

Library of Congress Control Number: 2021944559

Content Strategist: Humayra R. Khan
Content Development Specialist: Akanksha Marwah
Publishing Services Manager: Deepthi Unni
Project Manager: Sindhuraj Thulasingam
Design Direction: Brian Salisbury

Printed in the United States of America

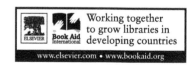

Working together
to grow libraries in
developing countries

www.elsevier.com • www.bookaid.org

Last digit is the print number: 9   8   7   6   5   4   3   2

Easy EMG

CONTENTS

PREFACE

We realize that many residents struggle with learning the basics of electrodiagnostic testing. We hope that this book provides a foundation that is easy to understand. This is not meant to be a comprehensive text. It is meant, rather, to serve as a bridge to more in-depth textbooks.

This third edition includes updates and additional chapters. In addition, we hope that the video clips will clarify the technical aspect of electrodiagnostic testing. The first three chapters are introductory in nature. They briefly review what electromyography (EMG) testing is and why we do it. Chapter 4 assesses nerve conduction studies. The needle portion of the examination is discussed in Chapter 5. Chapter 6 reviews the effects of injuries on peripheral nerves. Suggestions on how to plan out the examination are reviewed in Chapter 7. Chapter 8 examines some of the pitfalls that all electromyographers should recognize.

Chapters 9 through 20 review some of the commonly encountered clinical entities that the beginning electromyographer might encounter. Chapter 24 gives suggestions on how to write a complete electrodiagnostic report. Chapter 25 details the commonly accepted normal values for electrodiagnostic laboratory tests. It should be stressed, however, that each laboratory should develop its own set of normals based on its own particular patient population and electrodiagnostic equipment. Reimbursement issues are discussed in Chapter 26.

It should be noted that this book does not represent the complete spectrum of electrodiagnostic testing. Since this book is specifically targeted at novices in the field, some of the more complex testing, including somatosensory evoked potentials, blink reflex, and single-fiber EMG, is not discussed.

Although this text does review a great deal of technical information, the most important lesson one can learn, which is stressed repeatedly throughout the text, is that the electrodiagnostic test is an extension of the history and physical examination. We are physicians, first and foremost, with obligations to provide our patients with compassionate and quality care. We hope this book inspires lifelong learning.

Lyn D. Weiss MD
Jay M. Weiss MD
Julie K. Silver MD

The authors would like to dedicate this book to our teachers, to our mentors, and especially to our students.

Jay and Lyn Weiss want to thank the people who have taught us the most about what is important in life—our children (Ari, Lauren, Helene, Kyle, Stefan, Becca, Rachel, Benjamin, Olivia, Levon, Evelyn, and Mason).

VIDEO TABLE OF CONTENTS

CHAPTER 1

What Is an EMG?

Julie K. Silver

Electrodiagnostic studies seem confusing at first. Remember this: the entire purpose of electrodiagnostic studies is to help you figure out whether there is a problem with nerves, muscles, or both, and if so, where the problem is occurring (Fig. 1.1). The American Association of Neuromuscular and Electrodiagnostic Medicine uses the term *electrodiagnostic medicine* (which is sometimes abbreviated to EDX) to define the medical subspecialty that utilizes neurophysiologic techniques to diagnose, evaluate, and treat patients who are believed to have or who have documented physical impairments of the nervous, neuromuscular, and/or muscular systems.

We all recognize that the nervous system is a complicated part of our anatomy. Indeed, many medical students, residents, and fellows find their initial exposure to these tests and the courses in which they are taught overwhelming. However, the truth is that they are fairly straightforward and easy to understand.

If you do not believe this, think back to when you were a small child learning to read. At first, all of the letters in the alphabet did not make sense. Some had loops, some had straight lines, some had angled lines, and some had all of these. However, once you figured out all the letters, suddenly you could look at them anywhere and they made sense to you. Of course, you still could not read; that came later. Even after you learned the alphabet, the higher-level task of reading (at some point not too long after you learned the alphabet) eventually became a breeze. So, too, will electrodiagnostic studies become a breeze.

Think of the first half of this book as learning the alphabet. You will need to simply memorize some terms and try to understand when to use them and in which context they are meaningful—just like the alphabet letters. The second half of this book is the part where you learn to read or to put the things you have memorized to use in a logical way so that when electrodiagnostic studies are ordered, you can understand what information is being conveyed and how to perform the study. Keeping with the alphabet/reading example, more advanced electrodiagnostic textbooks (and clinical experience under experienced electromyographers) will teach you the equivalent of grammar and higher-level skills that are extremely important. Nevertheless, you do not need to know all that at first. Go through every chapter in this book, and just like you learned the alphabet and then learned to read, you will begin to become literate in electrodiagnostic studies—only it will happen much faster this time!

The term *electrodiagnostic studies* really encompasses a lot of different tests. The most common tests done (and the ones that will be presented in this book) are nerve conduction studies (NCS) and electromyography (EMG). Often people refer to *both* NCS and EMG as *just* EMG because these two tests are nearly always done together. But when you are talking with people who are familiar with electrodiagnostic testing, to avoid confusion it is best to speak of and write about (especially in your medical record documentation) these components separately. The tests can provide different information; however, both tests assess the electrical functioning of nerves and/or muscles.

It is interesting to note that electrodiagnostic studies originated in the 19th century but have been used consistently only within the past 30 to 40 years. This is because the machines became

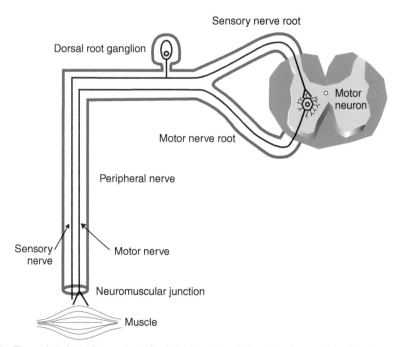

Fig. 1.1 The goal of electrodiagnostic studies is to determine whether there is a problem along the peripheral nervous system pathway and/or in the muscles and, if so, where the problem is. Examples of locations of possible lesions and associated diagnoses include:

Motor nerve cell body (anterior horn cell): amyotrophic lateral sclerosis
Root: cervical or lumbar radiculopathy
Axon: toxic neuropathy
Myelin: Guillain–Barré syndrome
Neuromuscular junction: myasthenia gravis
Muscle: muscular dystrophy

more sophisticated with computerization and, at the same time, easier to use. Highly refined techniques enhanced diagnostic applications and encouraged people to use these tests.

One of the things that will make it much easier for you to learn both EMG and NCS is to understand that *they are really extensions of the neurologic and musculoskeletal examination.* The more you know about the basic anatomy of the nerves and muscles, the easier it will be for you to learn about electrodiagnostic studies. If you are just beginning to learn about which nerves supply which muscles, this will be a slightly more complicated subject, but still very manageable. Just keep reading.

Table 1.1 is a summary of the process of performing electrodiagnostic studies. The rest of this chapter is devoted to explaining the two basic tests: EMG and NCS. You will simply need to memorize some of this; but hopefully, as you read, it will start to make sense.

Nerve Conduction Studies

NCS are done by placing electrodes on the skin and stimulating the nerves through electrical impulses (Fig. 1.2). To study motor nerves, electrodes are placed over a muscle that receives its innervation from the nerve you want to test (stimulate). The electrical response of the muscle is then recorded, and you can determine both how fast and how well the nerve responded. This

TABLE 1.1 ■ The Electrodiagnostic Process

1. Evaluate the patient by doing a history and physical examination, with the goal of developing a differential diagnosis.
2. Select the appropriate electrodiagnostic tests you want to perform to rule in or out diagnoses on your list.
3. Explain to the patient what the test will feel like and why it is being done.
4. Perform the study in a technically competent fashion, usually starting with NCS and then proceeding with EMG.
5. Interpret the results to arrive at the correct diagnosis or to narrow your list of differential diagnoses.
6. Communicate the test results to the referring physician in a timely and meaningful manner.

EMG, Electromyography; *NCS,* nerve conduction studies.

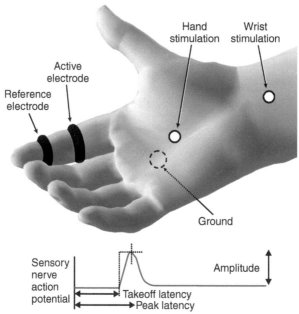

Fig. 1.2 This is the basic setup for a sensory nerve conduction study. The machine gives a tracing of the sensory nerve action potential (SNAP). The amplitude and latency can be measured easily.

is very valuable information and can help you determine whether the patient's condition is stemming from a problem with the nerve or with the muscle.

NCS are broken down into two categories: *motor* and *sensory* nerve conduction testing. The autonomic nervous system can be tested, but it rarely has clinical applications and is beyond the scope of this text. NCS can be performed on any *accessible* nerve, including peripheral nerves and cranial nerves.

The basic findings are generally twofold: (1) How fast is the impulse traveling (e.g., How well is the electrical impulse conducting?)? And (2) What does the electrical representation of the nerve stimulation (action potential morphology) look like on the screen (e.g., Does there appear to be a problem with the shape or height that might suggest an injury to some portion of the nerve, such as the axons or the myelin?)?

The terms you need to memorize in NCS are listed in Table 1.2. EMG terms are listed and explained in Chapter 5, Electromyography.

TABLE 1.2 ▪ Nerve Conduction Study Terms

Action potential: This is the waveform you see on the screen. (To give more details about what you are describing, more specific terms may include compound nerve action potential, compound motor action potential, or sensory nerve action potential.)

Amplitude: The maximal height of the action potential.

Antidromic: When the electrical impulse travels in the opposite direction of normal physiologic conduction (e.g., conduction of a motor nerve electrical impulse away from the muscle and toward the spine).

Conduction velocity: How fast the fastest part of the impulse travels (can also be referred to as a motor conduction velocity or a sensory conduction velocity).

F-wave: A compound muscle action potential evoked by antidromically stimulating a motor nerve from a muscle using maximal electrical stimulus. It represents the time required for a stimulus to travel antidromically toward the spinal cord and to return orthodromically to the muscle along a very small percentage of the fibers.

Latency: The time interval between the onset of a stimulus and the onset of a response (can also be referred to as a motor latency or a sensory latency).

H-reflex: A compound muscle action potential evoked by orthodromically stimulating sensory fibers, synapsing at the spinal level and returning orthodromically via motor fibers. The response is thought to be due to a monosynaptic spinal reflex (Hoffmann reflex) found in normal adults in the gastrocnemius–soleus and flexor carpi radialis muscles.

Orthodromic: When the electrical impulse travels in the same direction as normal physiologic conduction (e.g., when a motor nerve electrical impulse is transmitted toward the muscle and away from the spine, or when a sensory impulse travels toward the spine).

Electromyography

EMG is the process by which an examiner puts a needle into a particular muscle and studies the electrical activity of that muscle. This electrical activity comes from the muscle itself—no shocks are used to stimulate the muscle. EMG also differs from NCS because it does not involve actually testing nerves. However, you do get information about the nerves indirectly by testing the muscles. (Remember that all muscles are supplied by nerves, so if you can identify which muscles are affected by a disease process, then you simultaneously obtain information about the nerves that supply those muscles.)

So the EMG is different from NCS in the following ways:

1. In EMG, you use a needle and put it into the muscle rather than placing electrodes on the skin (NCS).
2. In EMG, you do not use any electrical shocks; rather, you are looking at the *intrinsic* electrical activity of the muscle.
3. In EMG, you get *direct* information about the muscles and *indirect* information about the nerves that supply the muscles you test.

CHAPTER 2

Why Perform Electrodiagnostic Studies?

Julie K. Silver

Electrodiagnostic testing is an important method for physicians and other healthcare profession-als to distinguish among many nerve and muscle disorders. One of the ways to think of electromy-ography (EMG) and nerve conduction studies (NCS) is to consider them pieces of a puzzle. The puzzle may be complicated with many pieces, or fairly straightforward with few pieces needed to solve it. To understand what you are seeing, whether it is a real puzzle or a figurative medical puz-zle, the more pieces you can put into place, the clearer the picture becomes. In medicine, some of the other puzzle pieces are the history, physical examination, laboratory tests, and imaging studies.

An important thing to remember is that electrodiagnostic studies represent a *physiologic* piece of the diagnostic puzzle. For example, unlike an magnetic resonance imaging (MRI) or an x-ray, which one can think of as sophisticated photographs, EMG and NCS provide information in real time about what is occurring physiologically with respect to the nerve and the muscle. This is not to say that imaging studies are not useful, but rather to explain that these tests complement each other and that each has a role in helping establish the correct diagnosis in neuromuscular disorders.

The take-home message is this: Electrodiagnostic studies are sometimes essential in establishing a par-ticular diagnosis and are sometimes not useful at all. As a clinician, it is important to understand when to recommend these studies, just as it is important to know when to order an imaging study. The more you learn about EMG and NCS, the more familiar you will become with their diagnostic usefulness.

In a practical sense, you can consider electrodiagnostic testing in any of the following circum-stances:

1. A patient is complaining of numbness.
2. A patient is complaining of tingling (paresthesias).
3. A patient has pain.
4. A patient has weakness.
5. A patient has a limp.
6. A patient has muscle atrophy.
7. A patient has depressed deep tendon reflexes.
8. A patient has fatigue.

Of course, it would be ridiculous to rely solely on any one of these signs or symptoms when recommending NCS and/or EMG. For example, a young woman comes in complaining of arm pain. The differential diagnosis should immediately include trauma as a source of the pain. Upon questioning you learn that in fact she fell, and on physical examination you note a large abrasion that explains her pain. To even consider electrodiagnostic studies in this situation is absurd. The point here is that a list of signs and symptoms does not lead you to automatically order electro-diagnostic studies. Rather, these tests can be thought of as *extensions of the history and physical examination* when someone has any one or more of the listed signs or symptoms that cannot be explained by the history and physical examination alone.

Clearly electrodiagnostic studies are useful to establish the correct diagnosis, but they are also useful to determine whether someone should have surgery and are often preferred over imaging studies when certain types of surgery are being considered. They are also done for prognostic reasons to follow the course of recovery (or deterioration) from an injury.

In summary, electrodiagnostic studies are used to:

1. Establish the correct diagnosis.
2. Localize the lesion.
3. Determine treatment even if the diagnosis is already known.
4. Provide information about the prognosis.

Consider the following examples:

Example 1

A man comes in with hand pain, paresthesias, and numbness that are most prominent in the index and long fingers. Upon questioning, he also reveals he has neck pain. The physical examination is inconclusive. The differential diagnosis includes carpal tunnel syndrome (median nerve compression at the wrist) and cervical radiculopathy. EMG and NCS are the studies of choice to establish the correct diagnosis.

Example 2

Another man comes in with the same symptoms, but he does not have neck pain. In the past, he was diagnosed with carpal tunnel syndrome and underwent an injection with local corticosteroid into the carpal tunnel, which completely alleviated his symptoms for a few months. (A good response to a corticosteroid injection in the carpal tunnel is both therapeutic and diagnostic for carpal tunnel syndrome.) Now, however, his symptoms are back with a vengeance. In this case of carpal tunnel syndrome, electrodiagnostic studies can be recommended to determine the severity of his condition and to help decide whether conservative management or surgery is the most appropriate course of treatment.

Example 3

A third man comes in; he had carpal tunnel surgery 3 months ago. His symptoms are much better, but he is still quite weak. Before his surgery he had EMG and NCS that demonstrated a very severe injury to the median nerve. Now he is a candidate for repeat electrodiagnostic studies to provide information about the prognosis. The new study can be compared to the old study, and information can be extrapolated about the current status of the median nerve and predicted future improvement.

The Skilled and Compassionate Electrodiagnostician

The reason you are reading this book is because skill matters. If you are going to perform electrodiagnostic studies on patients, you need to become an expert in electrodiagnostic medicine. The American Association of Neuromuscular and Electrodiagnostic Medicine (AANEM) provides information and recommendations on the qualifications for physicians and laboratory directors. For example, the AANEM recommends that physicians undergo at least 6 months of full-time supervised training during a physical medicine and rehabilitation (PM&R) or neurology residency or fellowship, and complete a minimum of 200 studies. To take the board examination offered by the American Board of Electrodiagnostic Medicine (ABEM), physicians must also have a minimum of 1 year's experience following their training. Reading this book, other textbooks, and journal articles, as well as studying anatomy in the context of electrodiagnostic medicine and performing a significant number of studies—at first with supervision and then on your own—will help turn you into an expert.

Even if electrodiagnostic studies become easy for you, they are not easy on your patients. Many patients are afraid to have electrodiagnostic studies. They may have heard that these tests are extremely painful, or they may have a genuine needle phobia. To get the information you need from these tests, it is important for you to be both technically skilled and able to put the patient at ease. The following suggestions will help lessen the patient's anxiety:

1. Avoid keeping the patient waiting, because that will only increase their anxiety.
2. Before you start, explain to the patient what you are going to do. Be sure the patient understands that the electrical stimulation occurs *only* with NCS and *not* with EMG.
3. Explain that these tests will be useful in determining the diagnosis.
4. Reassure the patient that you will stop the test at any point if they request you to do so. Be sure to honor that request should it occur.
5. Start with the area of greatest interest—especially if you suspect that the patient will not tolerate the entire study.
6. Although not typically used, analgesic or sedating medication can be given (particularly in pediatric patients).
7. During the test, distract the patient with conversation. It is usually easy to distract someone by asking them questions about what they like to do, where they like to go, and other similar questions. Some electromyographers play music of the patient's choosing during the test.
8. In most instances, it is best not to show patients the needle because many people associate more pain with a long needle rather than with a larger diameter. (The EMG needle is long, thin, and coated with Teflon, which moves through skin and muscle with less resistance, so it does not hurt as much as a larger-diameter conventional needle.) In addition, most patients feel more comfortable with the term *electrical stimulation* rather than *electrical shock*, which conjures up images of torture.
9. Assure the patient that you will minimize the length of the examination, doing only what is absolutely necessary to obtain the required information.
10. Keep the room warm. This serves two purposes. First of all, the patient is generally dressed in a gown and therefore is prone to being cold, so keeping the room warm will make them more comfortable. Second, the results of your electrodiagnostic test may be affected if the patient's extremity is cool (see Chapter 8, Pitfalls).

SPECIAL PRECAUTIONS

There are a number of clinical situations that deserve special mention. These are cases where electrodiagnostic studies can be safely done, as long as the physician takes measures to ensure the safety of the patient (and the physician) and the accuracy of the test.

Morbid Obesity

In patients who are overweight, it may be difficult (or impossible) to localize specific muscles. Care must be taken to ensure the needle is indeed placed in the appropriate muscle. Extra-long needles may be needed.

Thin Individuals

In thin patients, it is important not to insert the needle too far, because it can injure other tissues (e.g., a needle placed in the thoracic paraspinal muscles may penetrate the lung and cause a pneumothorax).

Bleeding Disorders

Individuals with known bleeding disorders or who are on anticoagulation therapy should be assessed on an individual basis and the risks and benefits of the test evaluated. It may be helpful to have recent laboratory testing for coagulation parameters. Therapeutic levels of anticoagulation are not a contraindication to EMG.

Blood Precautions

It is imperative to always practice safe needle-stick procedures to protect yourself and the patient from injury. These include always wearing gloves for the needle portion of the test, using a sterile disposable needle for the EMG, using a one-handed technique if needed for needle recapping, and immediately disposing of all sharps in an appropriate container.

CONTRAINDICATIONS

Strict contraindications to electrodiagnostic testing are relatively few. Obviously anyone who has a severe bleeding disorder or whose anticoagulation therapy is out of control should not undergo EMG. NCS are contraindicated in those with automatic implanted cardiac defibrillators. A patient with a cardiac pacemaker should not receive direct electrical stimulation over the pacemaker. Someone with an active skin or soft tissue infection (e.g., cellulitis) should not have a needle EMG anywhere near the infection.

COMPLICATIONS

Complications from electrodiagnostic studies are extremely rare when performed by a skilled clinician. Complications may include infection, bleeding, and accidental penetration of the needle into something other than the intended muscle (e.g., lung or nerves).

CONTROVERSY

As with nearly every test in medicine, there is controversy about when to do electrodiagnostic studies. There is no doubt that EMG and NCS provide valuable information and in many instances are worthwhile tests to pursue. However, they must be judiciously performed—as is the case with all medical testing. Of course, there would not be any controversy if these studies were painless, completely safe, and free, but this is not the case. They do cause some patient discomfort (although this can be minimized with a skilled and compassionate approach), and they are relatively expensive tests to perform.

Although these tests are generally safe, as with any injection there is a very small risk of complications. In instances where there is potential beneficial information from the test, then the risk–benefit ratio will fall in favor of performing the test. If the test is not realistically likely to be helpful in treatment then the risks (even if minimal) may outweigh the potential benefits.

The AANEM Recommended Policy For Electrodiagnostic Medicine note "minimum standards." First of these is the test should be medically indicated.[1] This would imply that the test would potentially enhance the patients care. Therefore it is important every time you consider performing electrodiagnostic studies to assess whether the test is necessary; whether it will help you determine the diagnosis, treatment, or prognosis of a patient's condition; and whether there is another test that might be less invasive and/or more cost-effective or that will provide the same information. It is important to always remember to *first do no harm*.

Reference

1. AANEM Recommended Policy For Electrodiagnostic Medicine. Approved by the American Association of Neuromuscular & Electrodiagnostic Medicine: September 1997; updated 1998, 1999, 2000, 2001, 2002, 2004, 2014, and 2017. Updated on November 2019.

CHAPTER 3

About the Machine

Julie K. Silver

The Basic Machine

Modern electrodiagnostic equipment consists of a computer and the associated hardware and software (Fig. 3.1). The hardware is fairly standard and typically includes a visual monitor, a keyboard, and computer hardware and software. The software varies in the same ways that all software varies—ease of use, ability to perform specific functions, and ability to interface with other software. However, all basic electrodiagnostic software allows the clinician:

- to perform both electromyography (EMG) and nerve conduction studies (NCS),
- to collect data,
- to analyze the results (through automatic calculations that are usually preprogrammed), and
- to store the information.

Data entry is done using a keyboard and/or a mouse. Machines have varying degrees of word processing functions and generation of reports through templates. When you are performing NCS, the information you need is displayed on a screen. During EMG studies, you will have the same visual screen information, but there also will be audio (sounds) that you will hear. Both the visual and the audio data are critical to properly interpreting EMG findings.

RECORDING ELECTRODES

It is important to understand electrode terms used in electrodiagnostic studies. Table 3.1 lists the common terms and in which studies they are used.

Surface Electrodes

Surface electrodes are used for routine NCS. The electrodes are typically either *ring* or *disk* electrodes (Fig. 3.2). They are also either *disposable* or *nondisposable*. The nondisposable electrodes are made of stainless steel, silver, or, rarely, gold that is soldered to multistrand conducting wires. These electrodes stick to the skin by using adhesive tape and can be reused. They should be cleaned between patients. It is necessary to use conducting gel with *nondisposable* electrodes to reduce impedance and prevent artifact (due to irregularities in the skin and the presence of hair follicles). *Disposable* electrodes have a sticky underside and a built-in conductive medium that allows them to adhere to the skin and to conduct electrical signals without the need for tape or gel.

Three surface electrodes are used in NCS: active and reference recording electrodes and ground electrodes. In EMG studies, surface electrodes are used for the ground and (in the case of a monopolar needle electrode) for the reference-recording electrode.

Needle Electrodes

Needle electrodes are generally reserved for EMG but are occasionally used in NCS. *Needle electrodes are disposable and are used only on one patient (one-time use).* Needle electrodes are classified as monopolar 3,3a, bipolar 3.3b, or concentric. Monopolar needles are typically less expensive, less

9

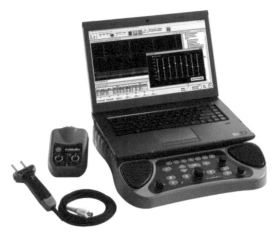

Fig. 3.1   Picture of an electromyography (EMG) machine. (Courtesy of Cadwell Laboratories.)

TABLE 3.1 ■ **Electrodes Used in NCS and EMG**

NCS
Active (surface electrode—this is also referred to as the pickup electrode)
Reference (surface electrode)
Ground (surface electrode)

EMG
Active (needle electrode)
Reference (surface electrode)[a]
Ground (surface electrode)

[a]A separate reference is used in EMG studies only if you are using a monopolar needle. Concentric needles
have a reference built into the needle, so there is no need for a separate reference.
EMG, Electromyography; *NCS*, nerve conduction studies.

---

painful (due to a narrower diameter and a Teflon coating on the shaft of the needle), and less electrically stable than bipolar or concentric needle electrodes. With a monopolar needle, you need a
separate surface reference electrode, whereas with a concentric needle, the reference is the barrel
of the needle and you do not need a separate surface reference electrode. There are also EMG
needles that allow for injections (e.g., botulinum toxin injections; see Fig. 3.3c). See Chapter 5,
Electromyography, for further description of the needles.

AMPLIFIERS

Amplifiers are very complicated parts of the electrodiagnostic machinery, but their concept is
fairly simple. *Amplifiers magnify the signal so that it can be displayed* (Fig. 3.4). Integrated circuits or
chips perform most amplification. *Preamplifiers* attenuate the biological signal before it ever gets
to the amplifier to (1) make sure that the filters have sufficient signal voltage to deal with and (2)
ensure that the level of signal voltage is much higher than that of system noise. The signal travels
first to the preamplifier, then to the filters, and then to the amplifier. The *differential* amplifier is
used extensively in electrodiagnostic studies, because it has the advantage of *common mode rejection*.
What this means is that unwanted signals are rejected rather than being amplified to the same

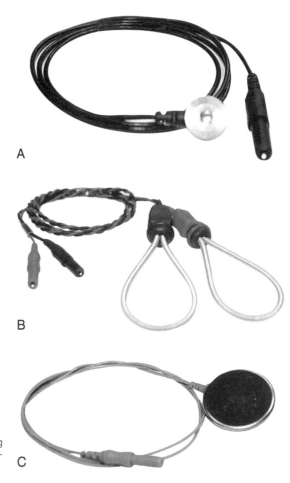

Fig. 3.2 (A) Disk electrode; (B) Ring electrode; (C) Ground electrode. (Courtesy of Cadwell Laboratories.)

A

B

C

degree as the biological signals that you are trying to study. The most common unwanted signal in the clinic is 60-Hz activity, which is caused by line voltage passing through electrical circuits.

The differential amplifier takes the electrical impulses from the active electrode and amplifies them. It then takes the impulses from the reference electrode, inverts them, and amplifies them. It then combines these two potentials. In this way, any common noise to both electrodes (extraneous electrical activity, distant myogenic noise, and EKG artifacts) is eliminated. Differences between the two electrodes, however, are amplified. This is the desired signal. Any common factors such as extraneous noise would be rejected, leading to the term *common mode rejection*. The common mode rejection ratio is a measure of how well an amplifier eliminates this type of common noise.

Filters

Filters are used to *faithfully reproduce the signal you want while trying to exclude both high- and low-frequency electrical noise*. All waveforms represent a summation of waves with different amplitudes, latencies, and frequencies. Every signal in both NCS and EMG passes through both a low-frequency and a high-frequency filter before being displayed. *Low-frequency* filters are called *high pass* because they let high-frequency signals pass through. The range at which there is

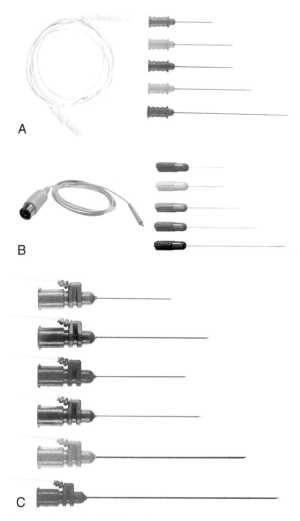

Fig. 3.3 (A) Photo of monopolar needle; (B) Photo of concentric needle; (C) Photo of an injectable needle. (Courtesy of Cadwell Laboratories.)

a cut-off of low-frequency signals depends on how you set the filter. Similarly, *high-frequency* filters are called *low pass* because they let low-frequency signals through. It is important to understand that there is always a trade-off when you use filters. The signal you want will be altered to some degree. For example, as the low-frequency filter is reduced, more low-frequency signals pass through and the duration of the recorded potential will be slightly longer. Likewise, if the high-frequency filter is decreased, more high-frequency signals are excluded and the latency of the recorded potential may be delayed. Table 3.2 summarizes the role of filters and gives the usual settings in NCS and EMG.

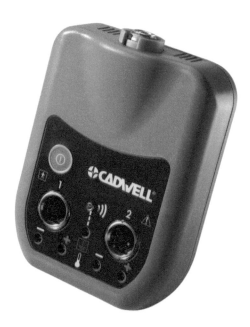

Fig. 3.4 Preamplifier. (Courtesy of Cadwell Laboratories.)

TABLE 3.2 ■ **Filters**

Low frequency	High pass	Filter out low-frequency signals that, if present, cause a wandering baseline
High frequency	Low pass	Filter out high-frequency signals that, if present, can obscure signals such as sensory nerve action potentials or fibrillation potentials and can cause a "noisy" baseline, especially on sensory studies

Display System

Display systems for electrodiagnostic studies are via a video computer screen. There are two settings on the display system with which you must be acquainted: the *sweep speed* and *sensitivity* (also sometimes called the *gain*). The primary purpose of adjusting the sweep speed and sensitivity is so that you can optimally see the signal displayed on the screen. The *horizontal* axis is the *sweep speed* and is shown in milliseconds (msec). There are 1000 msec in a second (Fig. 3.5). The *vertical* axis is the *sensitivity*, and this represents response amplitude (millivolts [mV] in motor studies and microvolts [µV] in sensory studies; Fig. 3.6). There are 1000 µV in a mV and 1000 mV in a volt (V). Suggested motor NCS settings are listed in Table 3.3. The initial settings for sensory NCS are listed in Table 3.4.

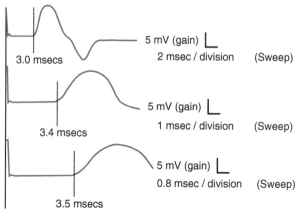

Fig. 3.5 Effects of latency with changes in sweep speed. (Adapted from Preston DC, Shapiro BE. *Electromyography and Neuromuscular Disorders*. London: Butterworth-Heinemann; 1998.)

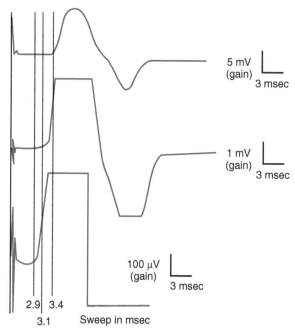

Fig. 3.6 Effect of increasing the sensitivity (gain) of a compound muscle action potential (CMAP). (Adapted from Preston DC, Shapiro BE. *Electromyography and Neuromuscular Disorders*. London: Butterworth-Heinemann; 1998.)

TABLE 3.3 ■ Initial Motor NCS Settings

Sweep speed	2–3 msec/division
Sensitivity (gain)	5000 µV/division (this means the same as 5 millivolts, 5 mV, or 5000 microvolts)
Low-frequency filter	10 Hz
High-frequency filter	10 kHz

NCS, Nerve conduction studies.
Adapted from Misulis K. *Essentials of Clinical Neurophysiology*. London: Butterworth-Heinemann; 1997.

TABLE 3.4 ▪ **Initial Sensory NCS Settings**

Sweep speed	1–2 msec/division—generally 10 divisions are present in a horizontal screen.
Sensitivity (gain)	20 μV/division
Low-frequency filter	2–10 Hz
High-frequency filter	2 kHz

NCS, Nerve conduction studies.
Adapted from Misulis K. *Essentials of Clinical Neurophysiology*. London: Butterworth-Heinemann; 1997.

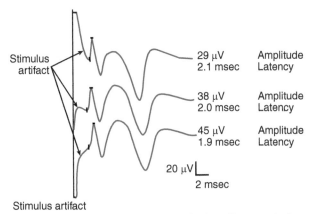

Fig. 3.7 Large stimulus artifact may falsely decrease the amplitude and increase the latency. (Adapted from Preston DC, Shapiro BE. *Electromyography and Neuromuscular Disorders*. London: Butterworth-Heinemann; 1998.)

ARTIFACTS AND TECHNICAL FACTORS

Stimulus Artifact

This is an electrically recorded response that is elicited directly from the stimulator. It occurs in all NCS; however, it only becomes a problem when the trailing edge of the recorded artifact overlaps with the potential being recorded (Fig. 3.7). Making sure the ground is between the recording and stimulating electrodes can minimize stimulus artifact.

Filters

Filters were discussed earlier in this chapter, but they are mentioned here because they can significantly contribute to the quality of your study. It is important to remember that the role of filters is *to faithfully reproduce the signal you want while trying to exclude both high- and low-frequency electrical noise.* The better the ratio of the recorded biologic signal to the unwanted electrical noise (signal-to-noise ratio, or s/n ratio), the clearer the electrical tracing and the more accurate the recorded potentials.

Electrode Placement

There are many issues that occur when electrodes are improperly placed. This discussion will be detailed throughout the rest of the book. Suffice it to say here that proper electrode placement is a critical part of performing accurate electrodiagnostic studies.

STIMULATION

An important concept in NCS is to understand *supramaximal stimulation*. The bottom line is this: nearly all measurements made in NCS are done with the assumption that the *strength* of the stimulus is high enough to depolarize every axon in the nerve (H-reflexes being a notable exception). This is achieved by gradually increasing the stimulus strength until you reach the point where the amplitude of the waveform is no longer increasing. That is the point of supramaximal stimulation. If supramaximal stimulation is not achieved at a distal site, then you might mistakenly interpret this recording as signifying axonal loss due to the low amplitude. At a proximal site, this might appear to be *conduction block* (failure of an action potential to be conducted past a particular point, whereas conduction is possible below the point of the block). In both instances, anomalous innervation or nerve injury may be suspected incorrectly.

Of course, the old adage "too much of a good thing is not good" applies to many things in life. When it comes to stimulation in NCS, too much stimulation may cause co-stimulation of adjacent nerves or may stimulate nerves farther from the site (falsely lowering the latency). So, the goal is to reach supramaximal stimulation without applying so much stimulation that adjacent nerves are also stimulated.

MEASUREMENTS

The machine will do most of the calculations for you, but you still need to measure the distance between stimulations and between the stimulation and the recording electrode when you are determining the conduction velocity. It is imperative that the measurements are done accurately. Other than a simple oversight of not correctly recording the distance with your tape measure, measurement errors can occur across joints if the patient's limb is moved in different positions, which changes the distance you are measuring. This commonly occurs in ulnar nerve studies when the elbow is straight and then becomes flexed. Therefore, during an ulnar nerve study, it is best to keep the elbow flexed and in the same position for the duration of that particular study (and at the same angle on both sides). Skin measurements are major sources of error in electrodiagnostic studies. This can be minimized by increasing the distance of the nerve segment being studied (i.e., the shorter the distance, the greater the effect of a measurement error). In general, when measuring distance, follow the course of the nerve rather than measuring the shortest distance between the stimulating and recording electrodes.

Besides a tape measure, another necessary measurement device in an electrodiagnostic lab is a thermometer. This is generally an infrared thermometer or a contact thermometer on the skin, which records the skin temperature. Abnormally cold extremities can falsely increase latencies and alter (generally increase) amplitudes, particularly of sensory nerves.

SWEEP SPEED AND SENSITIVITY

Both the sweep speed and sensitivity can affect your NCS results. As the sensitivity is increased, the onset latency will decrease. So, it is important to record all of your latency measurements using the same sensitivity and sweep speed.

CHAPTER 4

Nerve Conduction Studies

Lyn D. Weiss ▪ Jay M. Weiss

Nerve conduction studies (NCS) can be defined as the recording of a peripheral neural impulse at some location distant from the site where a propagating action potential is induced in a peripheral nerve. In other words, a nerve is stimulated at one or more sites along its course, and the electrical response of the nerve is recorded.

Whether or not a nerve is injured can be evaluated by testing the ability of the nerve to conduct an electrical impulse. NCS allow us to accurately localize focal lesions or allow us to detect generalized disease processes along accessible portions of the peripheral nervous system. The reliability of a study is increased when the technical aspects of the study are standardized. This chapter will review why it can be helpful to use NCS and how to perform them.

The NCS most commonly performed are compound muscle action potentials (CMAPs) for motor nerves, sensory nerve action potentials (SNAPs) for sensory nerves, compound nerve action potentials (CNAPs) for mixed (sensory and motor) nerves, and late responses (primarily F-waves and H-reflexes). For a discussion of F-waves and H-reflexes, see Chapter 12, Radiculopathy.

Physiology

When performing NCS, it is important to understand nerve physiology. After all, nerve studies are physiological, not anatomic, tests. To test nerve function, we must understand how nerves conduct signals.

Nerves conduct impulses through a traveling wave of depolarization along their axons. The axon is the peripheral extension of the proximally located nerve cell body. The cell body is located in the spinal cord for motor nerves (anterior horn cell) and peripherally in the dorsal root ganglion for sensory nerves (Fig. 4.1). The surface membrane surrounding the axon is called the axolemma, and the axoplasm is contained within the axon. At rest, the axon has an intracellular potential that is negative in relation to the extracellular potential. When an axon is conducting an electrical impulse, voltage-dependent channels open and allow an influx of sodium (Na^+) ions. This influx of positive ions depolarizes the axon; changes the resting potential further down the axon, causing those channels to open; and thus creates a wave of depolarization (Fig. 4.2).

While nerves have a physiological direction (from the spine in the case of motor nerves, and to the spine in the case of sensory nerves), if a nerve is electrically stimulated anywhere along its course, waves of depolarization will travel in both directions from that point. Nerve conduction can be measured orthodromically (physiological direction of nerve conduction) or antidromically (opposite to the physiological direction). Motor and sensory nerve action potentials can be measured through skin electrodes if the nerve is sufficiently superficial. It is more common (and technically easier) to measure motor nerves by recording electrical activity from the muscle it innervates.

As a rule, a NCS is done only on myelinated nerve fibers, because unmyelinated fibers conduct extremely slowly and do not contribute significantly to the CMAPs and SNAPs. A myelinated nerve fiber is composed of an axon and its surrounding myelin sheath (Fig. 4.3). Myelin is a connective covering surrounding motor nerve axons and many sensory nerve axons. Myelin is

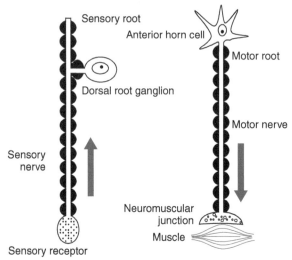

Fig. 4.1   Cell body of sensory and motor nerves.

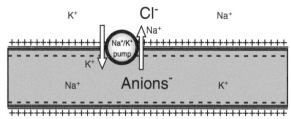

Fig. 4.2   Wave of depolarization.

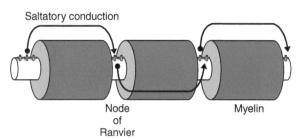

Fig. 4.3   Myelinated nerve.

produced by Schwann cells and functions to greatly increase the speed of nerve conduction. Myelin acts as an excellent insulator and permits saltatory conduction. This occurs when depolarization takes place only at the nodes between the myelin sheaths (referred to as nodes of Ranvier). For this reason, myelinated axons have their voltage-dependent sodium channels concentrated around the nodes, with few in the internodal regions. This type of *jumping* (or saltatory) conduction, where time is not required to depolarize axons between the nodes, permits a greater than tenfold increase in velocity.

Velocities in myelinated axons range from 40 to 70 m/sec. Unmyelinated axons, in contrast, are much slower—in the range of 1 to 5 m/sec. Unmyelinated axons do not conduct through saltatory conduction but have voltage-dependent channels located uniformly throughout the nerve. The speed of nerve conduction is largely contingent upon the amount of time it takes for voltage-dependent channels to open. Because unmyelinated nerves have a far greater number of channels per length of nerve, they conduct at less than one-tenth the speed of a myelinated nerve.

The most important points to remember about myelin are:

- Myelin helps nerves propagate an action potential faster.
- The myelin sheath functions as insulator of the axon.
- In myelinated nerves, depolarization occurs only at areas devoid of myelin (nodes of Ranvier), resulting in saltatory conduction.
- Conduction velocity is directly related to internodal length and efficiency of myelin insulation.

A demyelinated axon is a myelinated nerve that has lost its myelin covering. This does not become an unmyelinated nerve. While an unmyelinated axon can conduct an impulse slowly along its entire length, a demyelinated axon may not be able to conduct across a demyelinated area (as the sodium and potassium channels are only located near the nodes of Ranvier). This loss of conduction across a lesion is referred to as conduction block. The term *neurapraxia* is used to describe a lesion where conduction block is present (Figs. 4.4 and 4.5).

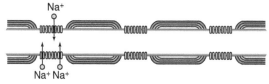

Normal axon and distribution of myelin

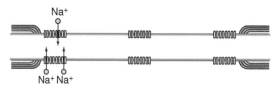

Injury to myelin
Note: A demyelinated axon does not become an unmyelinated axon

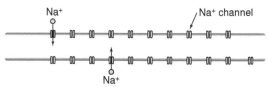

Unmyelinated axon
Note: Uniform distribution of sodium (Na+) channels in
unmyelinated axon compared to demyelinated axon

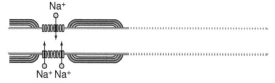

Injury to axon

Fig. 4.4 Types of nerve injuries.

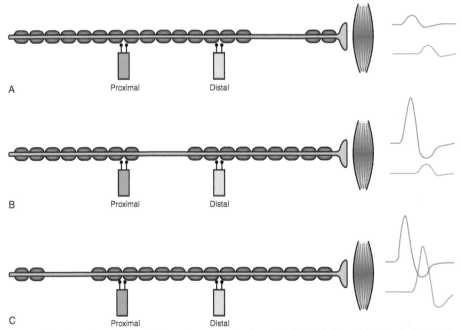

Fig. 4.5 Location of conduction block and nerve conduction study (NCS) findings. (A) lesion is distal to the distal stimulation; (B) lesion is between the proximal and distal stimulation; (C) lesion is proximal to the proximal stimulation. (From Preston DC, Shapiro BE. *Electromyography and Neuromuscular Disorders: Clinical-Electrophysiologic Correlations*. 2nd ed. Elsevier; 2005:42, fig. 3–19.)

It is important to note that while axons have an "all or none" response, an action potential represents the summation of many axons. Thus, a neurapraxic lesion can result in an amplitude decrement from less than 1% to nearly 100%. In reality, neurapraxic lesions of less than 20% are rarely diagnosed due to the amplitude differences normally seen from different sites of stimulation.

After a demyelinating lesion, as part of the recovery phase, there is typically regeneration of immature myelin. This immature myelin will not insulate as well as mature myelin, and therefore during NCS you may see a return of conduction but at a slower than normal velocity. Therefore, conduction slowing and conduction block are indicative of demyelinating, but not axonal lesions.

The Action Potential

The action potential is a summation of many potentials. In a CMAP, it is the summation of motor units (muscle fibers) that are firing, while a SNAP is a summation of individual sensory nerve fibers, each with its own amplitude and slightly different conduction velocity. This summation yields a characteristic (usually bell-shaped) curve. The part of the curve that begins to rise first represents components from the fastest fibers. The typical action potential is shown on a time versus amplitude chart (Fig. 4.6). The amplitude can be measured from onset to peak (A–B) or from peak to trough (B–C). The duration is the time from the onset to recovery (A–D). The area under the curve is a function of the amplitude and the duration. Instead of relying solely on amplitude, some electromyographers consider the area under the curve (measurement of the total area from negative departure from baseline to return to baseline) as a more accurate estimate of the number of axons firing. (Although this may seem a bit counterintuitive, it is important to remember that in electrodiagnostic terminology, *negative* refers to an upward deflection from baseline, and *positive* refers to a downward deflection from baseline.)

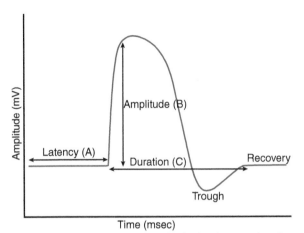

Fig. 4.6 Compound muscle action potential (latency, amplitude, duration, trough and recovery).

COMPONENTS OF THE ACTION POTENTIAL

Latency

The latency (4.6A) represents the time it takes from stimulation of the nerve to the beginning of the SNAP or the CMAP. In a CMAP, the onset latency represents the arrival time (at the recording electrode over the muscle) of the fastest-conducting nerve fibers. There is normal variation in the conduction velocity of the individual nerve fibers, producing a temporally dispersed curve. This is usually a gaussian or bell-shaped curve representing the number of fibers (amplitude) and how fast they are traveling (latency).

In sensory nerves, the latency is solely dependent on the speed of conduction of the fastest fibers and the distance the wave of depolarization travels. In motor nerves, in addition to the speed of the nerve and the distance traveled, the latency is also dependent on the amount of time it takes to synapse at the neuromuscular junction and the speed of intramuscular conduction. While the delay at the synapse or neuromuscular junction is typically brief (estimated to be approximately 1 msec), the exact duration can vary. Usually the latency is measured to the negative (upward) departure from baseline. If an initial positive departure is seen, the electrodes usually require repositioning, because it is likely that the recording electrode is over a muscle not innervated by the nerve being stimulated.

It must be stressed that a latency measurement without a standardized or recorded distance is meaningless. For example, if a patient has a large hand, the standard distance of 8 cm for median motor latency may not allow you to stimulate above the wrist. If you stimulate at 10 cm, but do not record that you stimulated at a distance of 10 cm, it will appear that the patient has slowing of the median nerve across the wrist, because it will take longer to travel a farther distance. Normal latencies are listed in Chapter 25, Tables of Normals.

Conduction Velocity

Conduction velocity is how fast the nerve is propagating an action potential. It can be calculated by the formula:

$$\text{velocity} = \text{distance}/\text{time}$$

As stated earlier, sensory nerves do not have a myoneural junction. Therefore, conduction velocity can be calculated directly by measuring the time it takes (in milliseconds) for the propagated action potential to travel the measured distance (in centimeters). Because motor nerves do

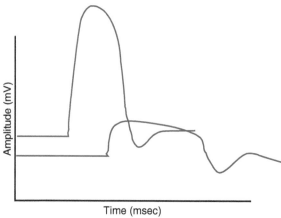

Fig. 4.7 Temporal dispersion.

conduct across a myoneural junction, the conduction velocity cannot be measured directly. Therefore, we use the formula:

$$velocity = change\ in\ distance/change\ in\ time$$

At least two sites must be stimulated. (The same nerve is stimulated both proximally and distally while recording over the same muscle.) The difference in distance from the two stimulation sites is then divided by the difference in latencies of the two action potentials obtained. Normal conduction velocities average above 50 m/sec in the upper extremities and above 40 m/sec in the lower extremities.

Amplitude

The amplitude (4.6B) of a CMAP represents the sum of the amplitudes of individual potentials. These individual potentials are generated by muscle fibers that are depolarized by nerve fiber axons of similar conduction velocities. The amplitude is therefore dependent on the integrity of the axons, the muscle fibers it depolarizes, and on the extent of variability of the conduction velocity of individual fibers. If some fibers are slow and others are fast, the action potential will be of longer duration (temporal dispersion) and lower amplitude (Fig. 4.7). When there is a CMAP with low amplitude, it is important to distinguish whether this is occurring because of temporal dispersion or a decreased number of axons (Fig. 4.8). The total area under the curve gives a better indication of the number of axons or muscle fibers depolarized than the amplitude itself, especially in cases of temporal dispersion.

In most cases, area measurements and amplitude measurements yield similar results, and either are used in common practice. Motor nerve amplitudes are measured in millivolts. Sensory nerve amplitudes are much smaller and are measured in microvolts. CMAP amplitude is most often measured from baseline to negative peak, but it also can be measured from peak to peak. SNAP amplitude is measured from negative peak to positive peak or from baseline to negative peak.

Duration

The duration (4.6C) is the time from the onset latency to the termination latency, in other words, the time from departure from baseline to final return to baseline. In some demyelinating diseases

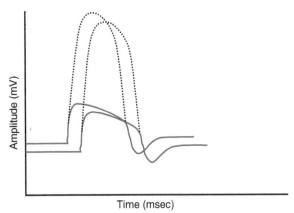

Time (msec)

Fig. 4.8   Axonal loss. Dotted line indicates normal amplitude.

with nerve fibers affected differently, the duration may be increased (temporal dispersion). Generally, temporal dispersion is seen in acquired neuropathies as opposed to congenital neuropathies.

TECHNICAL ASPECTS

Stimulators

A stimulator consists of two electrodes (a cathode and an anode). Generally, a handheld stimulator has a fixed distance between the two electrodes. When stimulating, in most cases the cathode (black or negative pole) is placed toward the direction in which the nerve is to be stimulated. The potential sites for stimulation are reviewed later in this chapter. Conduction gel should be used to ensure electrical contact. This may need to be reapplied periodically.

Sites of Stimulation

To accurately stimulate a nerve, it is necessary to know the anatomy of the nerve. Given a strong enough impulse, any nerve can be stimulated. The more superficial the nerve, the easier (and more accurate) stimulation becomes. In reality, nerves are usually stimulated when they are relatively superficial. This permits an electrical impulse that the patient can tolerate. Superficial stimulation also allows a more precise localization of the site on the nerve where it is stimulated. The farther away the nerve is from the cathode, the stronger the stimulus required. Supramaximal stimulation occurs when further increases in the intensity of the stimulus will not change the amplitude of the recorded potential. Increases beyond this point, however, can change the latency or stimulate adjacent nerves. Care should be taken not to *overstimulate*.

Some nerves may only be accessible to stimulation for a limited distance along the course of the nerve, whereas others can be stimulated at many sites along the nerve. In simple motor nerve studies, two stimulus sites may be used. In cases of suspected entrapment, it is important to be able to stimulate proximal and distal to the suspected area of involvement.

Recording Electrodes

Three electrodes are used to record each potential in NCS and electromyography. They are the active, reference, and ground electrodes.

Active (recording) electrode: The active or recording electrode should be placed over the muscle belly (preferably over the motor point, where the nerve enters the muscle) during motor studies. During sensory studies, the active (recording) electrode should be placed directly over the nerve (where the nerve is as superficial as possible).

Reference electrode: When attempting to record a CMAP, the reference electrode (sometimes called the E2 or G2) should be placed on a nearby tendon or bone away from the muscle. When performing SNAPs, it has been shown that 3 to 4 cm is the optimal interelectrode separation. If SNAP electrodes are placed too close to each other, decreased amplitude resembling an axonal lesion can occur. CMAPs are less affected than SNAPs when electrodes are placed less than 3 to 4 cm apart.

Ground electrode: The third type of electrode is called the ground electrode. Grounding is important to reduce artifact. Usually the ground is larger than the recording electrodes and provides a large surface area in contact with the patient. The ground electrode should be placed between the stimulating electrode and the recording electrode.

LATE RESPONSES

The H-reflex is a monosynaptic or oligosynaptic spinal reflex involving both motor and sensory fibers. It electrically tests some of the same fibers as are tested in the ankle jerk reflexes. In fact, it is rare to be unable to obtain an H-reflex in the presence of an ankle-jerk reflex. If this occurs, technical factors should be considered. In theory it is a sensitive measure in assessing radiculopathy because (1) it helps to assess proximal lesions, (2) it becomes abnormal relatively early in the development of radiculopathy, and (3) it incorporates sensory fiber function proximal to the dorsal root ganglion. The H-reflex primarily assesses afferent and efferent S1 fibers. Clinically, L5 and S1 radiculopathies may appear similar on electromyography (EMG) due to the overlap of myotomes. H-reflexes are probably of greatest value in distinguishing S1 from L5 radiculopathies.

When assessing for S1 radiculopathy, the H-reflex latency is recorded from the gastrocnemius–soleus muscle group upon stimulating the tibial nerve in the popliteal fossa (Fig. 4.9). The H-reflex is elicited with a submaximal stimulation with the cathode proximal to the anode. As the intensity of the stimulation is gradually increased from peak H-amplitude, we generally see a diminishment of the H-amplitude with a concurrent increase in the M-wave amplitude. With supramaximal stimulation, the H-reflex is usually absent.

The H-reflex can also be obtained by recording over the flexor carpi radialis muscle and stimulating the median nerve at the elbow. The median H-reflex is less commonly performed and clinically is less likely to be helpful for radiculopathy than a lower extremity H-reflex. Generally, gastrocnemius-soleus H-reflex latency side-to-side differences of greater than 1.5 msec are suggestive of S1 radiculopathy.

Although the H-reflex is sensitive, it has certain limitations:

1. Patients with S1 radiculopathy can have a normal H-reflex.
2. An abnormal H-reflex is only suggestive, but not definitive, for radiculopathy because the abnormality may originate in other components of the long pathway involved, such as the peripheral nerves, plexuses, or spinal cord.
3. Once the H-reflex becomes abnormal, it usually does not return to normal, even over time.
4. The H-reflex is often absent in otherwise normal individuals over the age of 60 years.

The reflexes therefore can be considered sensitive, but not specific, indicators of pathology. Latency of the H-reflex is dependent on the age and leg length of the patient (Table 4.1). A side-to-side amplitude difference of 60% or more may also indicate pathology.

F-waves are low-amplitude late responses thought to be due to antidromic activation of motor neurons (anterior horn cells) following peripheral nerve stimulation, which then cause orthodromic impulses to pass back along the involved motor axons. Some electromyographers have called this a *backfiring* of axons. It is called the F-wave because it was first noted in intrinsic foot muscles. The F-wave has a small amplitude, a variable configuration, and a variable latency. Generally, F-wave amplitudes are less than 5% of the orthodromically generated motor responses

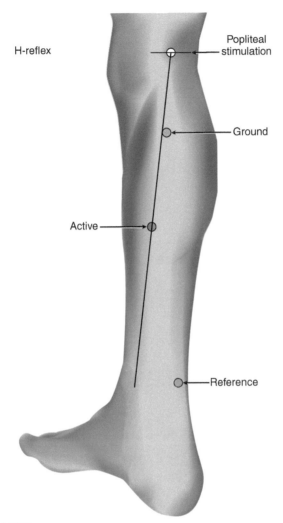

Fig. 4.9 Setup for H-reflex.

(M-responses), as most of the responses are extinguished at the spinal level. The most widely used parameter is the latency of the shortest reproducible response. The F-wave can be found in many muscles of the upper and lower extremities. Unfortunately, F-waves have not turned out to be valuable tests for radiculopathy as initially hoped. The reasons for this are:

1. The pathways involve only the motor fibers.
2. As with the H-reflex, it involves a long neuronal pathway so that if there is a focal lesion, it might be obscured.
3. If an abnormality is present, the F-wave will not pinpoint the exact location because any lesion, from the anterior horn cell to the muscle being tested, can affect the F-wave similarly.
4. Because muscles have multiple root innervations, the shortest latency may reflect the healthy fibers in the nonaffected root.

TABLE 4.1 ■ H-Reflex Values Based on Age and Height: (H = 2.74 + 0.05 × Age + 0.14 × Height + 1.4)

Height (cm)	Age (Years)															
	15	20	25	30	35	40	45	50	55	60	65	70	75	80	85	90
100	18.89	19.14	19.39	19.64	19.89	20.14	20.39	20.64	20.89	21.14	21.39	21.64	21.89	22.14	22.39	22.64
110	20.29	20.54	20.79	21.04	21.29	21.54	21.79	22.04	22.29	22.54	22.79	23.04	23.29	23.54	23.79	24.04
120	21.69	21.94	22.19	22.44	22.69	22.94	23.19	23.44	23.69	23.94	24.19	24.44	24.69	24.94	25.19	25.44
130	23.09	23.34	23.59	23.84	24.09	24.34	24.59	24.84	25.09	25.34	25.59	25.84	26.09	26.34	26.59	26.84
135	23.79	24.04	24.29	24.54	24.79	25.04	25.29	25.54	25.79	26.04	26.29	26.54	26.79	27.04	27.29	27.54
140	24.49	24.74	24.99	25.24	25.49	25.74	25.99	26.24	26.49	26.74	26.99	27.24	27.49	27.74	27.99	28.24
141	24.63	24.88	25.13	25.38	25.63	25.88	26.13	26.38	26.63	26.88	27.13	27.38	27.63	27.88	28.13	28.38
142	24.77	25.02	25.27	25.52	25.77	26.02	26.27	26.52	26.77	27.02	27.27	27.52	27.77	28.02	28.27	28.52
143	24.91	25.16	25.41	25.66	25.91	26.16	26.41	26.66	26.91	27.16	27.41	27.66	27.91	28.16	28.41	28.66
144	25.05	25.3	25.55	25.8	26.05	26.3	26.55	26.8	27.05	27.3	27.55	27.8	28.05	28.3	28.55	28.8
145	25.19	25.44	25.69	25.94	26.19	26.44	26.69	26.94	27.19	27.44	27.69	27.94	28.19	28.44	28.69	28.94
146	25.33	25.58	25.83	26.08	26.33	26.58	26.83	27.08	27.33	27.58	27.83	28.08	28.33	28.58	28.83	29.08
147	25.47	25.72	25.97	26.22	26.47	26.72	26.97	27.22	27.47	27.72	27.97	28.22	28.47	28.72	28.97	29.22
148	25.61	25.86	26.11	26.36	26.61	26.86	27.11	27.36	27.61	27.86	28.11	28.36	28.61	28.86	29.11	29.36
149	25.75	26	26.25	26.5	26.75	27	27.25	27.5	27.75	28	28.25	28.5	28.75	29	29.25	29.5
150	25.89	26.14	26.39	26.64	26.89	27.14	27.39	27.64	27.89	28.14	28.39	28.64	28.89	29.14	29.39	29.64
151	26.03	26.28	26.53	26.78	27.03	27.28	27.53	27.78	28.03	28.28	28.53	28.78	29.03	29.28	29.53	29.78
152	26.17	26.42	26.67	26.92	27.17	27.42	27.67	27.92	28.17	28.42	28.67	28.92	29.17	29.42	29.67	29.92
153	26.31	26.56	26.81	27.06	27.31	27.56	27.81	28.06	28.31	28.56	28.81	29.06	29.31	29.56	29.81	30.06
154	26.45	26.7	26.95	27.2	27.45	27.7	27.95	28.2	28.45	28.7	28.95	29.2	29.45	29.7	29.95	30.2
155	26.59	26.84	27.09	27.34	27.59	27.84	28.09	28.34	28.59	28.84	29.09	29.34	29.59	29.84	30.09	30.34
156	26.73	26.98	27.23	27.48	27.73	27.98	28.23	28.48	28.73	28.98	29.23	29.48	29.73	29.98	30.23	30.48
157	26.87	27.12	27.37	27.62	27.87	28.12	28.37	28.62	28.87	29.12	29.37	29.62	29.87	30.12	30.37	30.62
158	27.01	27.26	27.51	27.76	28.01	28.26	28.51	28.76	29.01	29.26	29.51	29.76	30.01	30.26	30.51	30.76
159	27.15	27.4	27.65	27.9	28.15	28.4	28.65	28.9	29.15	29.4	29.65	29.9	30.15	30.4	30.65	30.9
160	27.29	27.54	27.79	28.04	28.29	28.54	28.79	29.04	29.29	29.54	29.79	30.04	30.29	30.54	30.79	31.04
161	27.43	27.68	27.93	28.18	28.43	28.68	28.93	29.18	29.43	29.68	29.93	30.18	30.43	30.68	30.93	31.18
162	27.57	27.82	28.07	28.32	28.57	28.82	29.07	29.32	29.57	29.82	30.07	30.32	30.57	30.82	31.07	31.32
163	27.71	27.96	28.21	28.46	28.71	28.96	29.21	29.46	29.71	29.96	30.21	30.46	30.71	30.96	31.21	31.46
164	27.85	28.1	28.35	28.6	28.85	29.1	29.35	29.6	29.85	30.1	30.35	30.6	30.85	31.1	31.35	31.6
165	27.99	28.24	28.49	28.74	28.99	29.24	29.49	29.74	29.99	30.24	30.49	30.74	30.99	31.24	31.49	31.74
166	28.13	28.38	28.63	28.88	29.13	29.38	29.63	29.88	30.13	30.38	30.63	30.88	31.13	31.38	31.63	31.88

167	28.27	28.52	28.77	29.02	29.27	29.52	29.77	30.02	30.27	30.52	30.77	31.02	31.27	31.52	31.77	32.02
168	28.41	28.66	28.91	29.16	29.41	29.66	29.91	30.16	30.41	30.66	30.91	31.16	31.41	31.66	31.91	32.16
169	28.55	28.8	29.05	29.3	29.55	29.8	30.05	30.3	30.55	30.8	31.05	31.3	31.55	31.8	32.05	32.3
170	28.69	28.94	29.19	29.44	29.69	29.94	30.19	30.44	30.69	30.94	31.19	31.44	31.69	31.94	32.19	32.44
171	28.83	29.08	29.33	29.58	29.83	30.08	30.33	30.58	30.83	31.08	31.33	31.58	31.83	32.08	32.33	32.58
172	28.97	29.22	29.47	29.72	29.97	30.22	30.47	30.72	30.97	31.22	31.47	31.72	31.97	32.22	32.47	32.72
173	29.11	29.36	29.61	29.86	30.11	30.36	30.61	30.86	31.11	31.36	31.61	31.86	32.11	32.36	32.61	32.86
174	29.25	29.5	29.75	30	30.25	30.5	30.75	31	31.25	31.5	31.75	32	32.25	32.5	32.75	33
175	29.39	29.64	29.89	30.14	30.39	30.64	30.89	31.14	31.39	31.64	31.89	32.14	32.39	32.64	32.89	33.14
176	29.53	29.78	30.03	30.28	30.53	30.78	31.03	31.28	31.53	31.78	32.03	32.28	32.53	32.78	33.03	33.28
177	29.67	29.92	30.17	30.42	30.67	30.92	31.17	31.42	31.67	31.92	32.17	32.42	32.67	32.92	33.17	33.42
178	29.81	30.06	30.31	30.56	30.81	31.06	31.31	31.56	31.81	32.06	32.31	32.56	32.81	33.06	33.31	33.56
179	29.95	30.2	30.45	30.7	30.95	31.2	31.45	31.7	31.95	32.2	32.45	32.7	32.95	33.2	33.45	33.7
180	30.09	30.34	30.59	30.84	31.09	31.34	31.59	31.84	32.09	32.34	32.59	32.84	33.09	33.34	33.59	33.84
181	30.23	30.48	30.73	30.98	31.23	31.48	31.73	31.98	32.23	32.48	32.73	32.98	33.23	33.48	33.73	33.98
182	30.37	30.62	30.87	31.12	31.37	31.62	31.87	32.12	32.37	32.62	32.87	33.12	33.37	33.62	33.87	34.12
183	30.51	30.76	31.01	31.26	31.51	31.76	32.01	32.26	32.51	32.76	33.01	33.26	33.51	33.76	34.01	34.26
184	30.65	30.9	31.15	31.4	31.65	31.9	32.15	32.4	32.65	32.9	33.15	33.4	33.65	33.9	34.15	34.4
185	30.79	31.04	31.29	31.54	31.79	32.04	32.29	32.54	32.79	33.04	33.29	33.54	33.79	34.04	34.29	34.54
186	30.93	31.18	31.43	31.68	31.93	32.18	32.43	32.68	32.93	33.18	33.43	33.68	33.93	34.18	34.43	34.68
187	31.07	31.32	31.57	31.82	32.07	32.32	32.57	32.82	33.07	33.32	33.57	33.82	34.07	34.32	34.57	34.82
188	31.21	31.46	31.71	31.96	32.21	32.46	32.71	32.96	33.21	33.46	33.71	33.96	34.21	34.46	34.71	34.96
189	31.35	31.6	31.85	32.1	32.35	32.6	32.85	33.1	33.35	33.6	33.85	34.1	34.35	34.6	34.85	35.1
190	31.49	31.74	31.99	32.24	32.49	32.74	32.99	33.24	33.49	33.74	33.99	34.24	34.49	34.74	34.99	35.24
191	31.63	31.88	32.13	32.38	32.63	32.88	33.13	33.38	33.63	33.88	34.13	34.38	34.63	34.88	35.13	35.38
192	31.77	32.02	32.27	32.52	32.77	33.02	33.27	33.52	33.77	34.02	34.27	34.52	34.77	35.02	35.27	35.52
193	31.91	32.16	32.41	32.66	32.91	33.16	33.41	33.66	33.91	34.16	34.41	34.66	34.91	35.16	35.41	35.66
194	32.05	32.3	32.55	32.8	33.05	33.3	33.55	33.8	34.05	34.3	34.55	34.8	35.05	35.3	35.55	35.8
195	32.19	32.44	32.69	32.94	33.19	33.44	33.69	33.94	34.19	34.44	34.69	34.94	35.19	35.44	35.69	35.94
196	32.33	32.58	32.83	33.08	33.33	33.58	33.83	34.08	34.33	34.58	34.83	35.08	35.33	35.58	35.83	36.08
197	32.47	32.72	32.97	33.22	33.47	33.72	33.97	34.22	34.47	34.72	34.97	35.22	35.47	35.72	35.97	36.22
198	32.61	32.86	33.11	33.36	33.61	33.86	34.11	34.36	34.61	34.86	35.11	35.36	35.61	35.86	36.11	36.36
199	32.75	33	33.25	33.5	33.75	34	34.25	34.5	34.75	35	35.25	35.5	35.75	36	36.25	36.5

Continued

TABLE 4.1 ■ H-Reflex Values Based on Age and Height: (H = 2.74 + 0.05 × Age + 0.14 × Height + 1.4)—Cont'd

Height (cm)	Age (Years)															
	15	20	25	30	35	40	45	50	55	60	65	70	75	80	85	90
200	32.89	33.14	33.39	33.64	33.89	34.14	34.39	34.64	34.89	35.14	35.39	35.64	35.89	36.14	36.39	36.64
201	33.03	33.28	33.53	33.78	34.03	34.28	34.53	34.78	35.03	35.28	35.53	35.78	36.03	36.28	36.53	36.78
202	33.17	33.42	33.67	33.92	34.17	34.42	34.67	34.92	35.17	35.42	35.67	35.92	36.17	36.42	36.67	36.92
203	33.31	33.56	33.81	34.06	34.31	34.56	34.81	35.06	35.31	35.56	35.81	36.06	36.31	36.56	36.81	37.06
204	33.45	33.7	33.95	34.2	34.45	34.7	34.95	35.2	35.45	35.7	35.95	36.2	36.45	36.7	36.95	37.2
205	33.59	33.84	34.09	34.34	34.59	34.84	35.09	35.34	35.59	35.84	36.09	36.34	36.59	36.84	37.09	37.34
206	33.73	33.98	34.23	34.48	34.73	34.98	35.23	35.48	35.73	35.98	36.23	36.48	36.73	36.98	37.23	37.48
207	33.87	34.12	34.37	34.62	34.87	35.12	35.37	35.62	35.87	36.12	36.37	36.62	36.87	37.12	37.37	37.62
208	34.01	34.26	34.51	34.76	35.01	35.26	35.51	35.76	36.01	36.26	36.51	36.76	37.01	37.26	37.51	37.76
209	34.15	34.4	34.65	34.9	35.15	35.4	35.65	35.9	36.15	36.4	36.65	36.9	37.15	37.4	37.65	37.9
210	34.29	34.54	34.79	35.04	35.29	35.54	35.79	36.04	36.29	36.54	36.79	37.04	37.29	37.54	37.79	38.04
215	34.99	35.24	35.49	35.74	35.99	36.24	36.49	36.74	36.99	37.24	37.49	37.74	37.99	38.24	38.49	38.74
220	35.69	35.94	36.19	36.44	36.69	36.94	37.19	37.44	37.69	37.94	38.19	38.44	38.69	38.94	39.19	39.44
230	37.09	37.34	37.59	37.84	38.09	38.34	38.59	38.84	39.09	39.34	39.59	39.84	40.09	40.34	40.59	40.84

TABLE 4.2 ■ **Comparison of H-Reflexes and F-Waves**

Parameter	H-Reflex	F-Wave
Derivation of name	Originally described by Hoffmann	Originally obtained in foot muscles
Type of synapse	Monosynaptic or oligosynaptic	None (a backfiring of individual axons)
Pathway	Sensory orthodromic	Motor antidromic
	Motor antidromic	Motor orthodromic
Stimulus required	Submaximal (stronger stimulation produces inhibition secondary to collision of orthodromic impulses by antidromic conduction in motor axons)	Supramaximal
Where can they be elicited? (normals)	Soleus	Most muscles (distal preferred)
	Flexor carpi radialis	
Stimulation site	Posterior tibial nerve in popliteal fossa	Along peripheral nerve
Stimulus cathode	Proximal	Proximal
Size of response (compared to M)	Amplification of motor response centrally (due to reflex activation of motor neurons)	Small (motor neurons are activated infrequently with antidromic stimulation)
Facilitation	Enhanced by maneuvers that increase motor-neuron pool excitability (CNS lesion)	N/A
Uses	S1 radiculopathy (sensitive but not specific)	Demyelinating polyneuropathies
		Guillain–Barré syndrome
	Guillain–Barré syndrome	Proximal nerve or root injury (not test of choice; nonspecific)
Latency, amplitude, and configuration	Reproducible latency and configuration (amplitude dependent on stimulation)	Variable in amplitude, latency, and configuration
Side-to-side difference	>1.5 msec	>2 msec from hand
		>3 msec from calf
		>4 msec from foot
Ratio	N/A	$\dfrac{F-M-1}{2M}$

5. The latency and amplitude of an F-wave is variable so that multiple stimulations must be performed to find the shortest latency. If not enough stimulations are done (usually more than 10), the shortest latency may not be apparent. Thus, the use of F-waves in evaluating for radiculopathy is extremely limited and should not be the sole basis upon which the diagnosis is made. See Table 4.2 for a comparison of H-reflexes and F-waves.

According to the American Association of Neuromuscular and Electrodiagnostic Medicine, "the current body of evidence (substantiated by multiple studies published in well-respected peer-reviewed medical journals) does not support the use of F-waves in isolation to diagnose radiculopathy."[1]

F-Wave Ratio

Because errors can occur when measuring distances for F-wave conduction velocities, an alternative F-wave technique was developed that did not require distance measurements. The ratio is as follows:

$$\frac{(F - \text{wave latency} - CMAP \text{ latency}) - 1 \text{ msec}}{CMAP \text{ latency} \times 2}$$

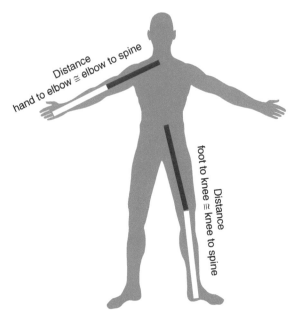

Fig. 4.10 F-wave ratios are calculated based on the assumption that the distance from the elbow (or knee) to the hand (or foot) is approximately equal to the distance from the elbow (or knee) to the spinal cord.

Substituting "M" for CMAP latency, this ratio may be rewritten as $(F - M - 1)/2M$. The ratio assumes that the distance from the elbow (or knee) to the hand (or foot) is approximately equal to the distance from the elbow (or knee) to the spinal cord (Fig. 4.10). Therefore, stimulation must be performed at the elbow or knee.

The normal F-wave ratio in the upper limb is approximately 1±0.3, and in the lower limb the normal F-ratio is 1.1±0.3. A ratio higher than 1.3 indicates a proximal lesion, because the numerator of the equation includes the proximal stimulation from the F-wave. A ratio below 0.7 indicates a distal lesion, because a larger CMAP latency will decrease the numerator and increase the denominator. Therefore, an F-ratio is not necessarily more sensitive than F-latency, but it does allow one to assess whether the slowing is in the proximal or distal segment of the nerve. It should be noted that F-waves are nonspecific. Therefore, interpreting NCS results using F-waves must be done in conjunction with other information.

Important Points to Remember

- When stimulating proximal and distal sites, the waveforms should be similar in morphology and duration. For motor studies, amplitude should not decrease by more than 20% on proximal stimulation (when compared to the distal amplitude). A notable exception to this 20% rule is the tibial nerve, where due to its depth, it frequently does not reach supramaximal stimulation in the popliteal fossa.
- Nonidentical waveforms may be secondary to accidental stimulation of another nerve. For example, the fibular and tibial nerves are very close in the popliteal fossa. If the pulse width (duration of the stimulus) is increased, the wrong nerve may be stimulated. Usually, the CMAP that results will have an initial positive (downward) deflection, because the active electrode is not over the muscle being stimulated. (If you are not sure which nerve is being stimulated, check for the physiological response. For example, if the ankle plantar flexes, the tibial nerve is usually being stimulated.)

TABLE 4.3 ■ Nerve Conduction Studies Setup

Nerve	Recording (Active) Electrode	Reference Electrode	Ground	Stimulation
Median: Motor (see Fig. A1.1 and Video 4.1)	Place on the anatomic center of the abductor pollicis brevis (usually about ½ the distance from the distal wrist crease to the metacarpal phalangeal joint).	Place on the proximal phalanx of the thumb. Place 3–4 cm distal to the recording electrode.	Place on the dorsum of the hand between the active electrode and the stimulator.	1. *Midwrist:* Distal stimulation is on the palmar surface of the hand between the tendons of the flexor carpi radialis and the palmaris longus. Stimulation should be 8 cm proximal to the active electrode. 2. *Elbow:* Stimulate proximal and medial to the antecubital space, just lateral to the brachial artery. 3. *Axilla:* Stimulation is performed in the axilla at least 10 cm proximal to the elbow stimulation.
Median: Sensory (antidromic) (see Fig. A1.2 and Video 4.2)	Place over the proximal interphalangeal joint on the second finger.	Place the reference electrode over the distal interphalangeal joint.	Ground is placed on the dorsum of the hand between the active electrode and stimulator.	The stimulation points occur 7 cm proximal to the active electrode at the midpalm, and 7 cm proximal to the midpalm at the wrist (between the tendons of the flexor carpi radialis and the palmaris longus). (For large hands, 8 cm can be used. For small hands, 6 cm can be used.)
Ulnar: Motor (see Fig. A1.3 and Video 4.3)	Place on the center of the abductor digiti minimi. It may help to palpate that muscle by abducting the fifth digit.	Place distally over the fifth digit.	Place on the dorsum of the hand between the active and the stimulating electrodes.	1. *Wrist:* Stimulate 8 cm proximally from the active electrode. This is usually just medial to the flexor carpi ulnaris tendon. 2. *Below the elbow:* When stimulating at the elbow region, you must flex the elbow so there is an angle of about 90 degrees. Feel for the ulnar groove (the funny bone) and stimulate just below this area. 3. *Above the elbow:* The stimulation site is located at least 10 cm proximal to the below elbow stimulation in line with the path of the ulnar nerve. 4. *Axilla:* This stimulation site is located at least 10 cm proximal to the above elbow site at about the midpoint of the arm in the axilla.

Remember that the arm should be maintained with the same elbow flexion when stimulating and measuring the nerve.

The responses from all four sites should be similar in waveform, amplitude, and duration.

Continued

TABLE 4.3 ■ Nerve Conduction Studies Setup—Cont'd

Nerve	Recording (Active) Electrode	Reference Electrode	Ground	Stimulation
Dorsal ulnar cutaneous nerve (see Fig. A1.4 and Video 4.4)	Place on the dorsum of the hand, between the fourth and fifth metacarpal bones.	Place at the base of the fifth digit.	Place on the dorsum of the hand between the active and stimulating electrodes.	Place about 10 cm proximal to the recording electrode (active electrode slightly proximal to the ulnar styloid). The hand should be pronated.
Ulnar: Sensory (antidromic) (see Fig. A1.5 and Video 4.5)	Place on the fifth digit over the proximal interphalangeal joint (PIP) joint.	Place over the fifth distal interphalangeal (DIP) joint, so that a distance of not less than 3 cm is maintained.	Place on the dorsum of the hand between the active and stimulating electrodes.	Stimulate at the wrist a distance of 14 cm proximal from the active electrode near the proximal crease of the wrist.
Radial: Sensory (antidromic) (see Fig. A1.6 and Video 4.6)	Place over the sensory branch as it crosses the extensor pollicis longus tendon. This can be palpated on the ulnar side of the anatomic snuffbox when the thumb is extended.	Place on the lateral side of the head of the second metacarpal about 3–4 cm distal to the active electrode.	Place between the active electrode and the stimulating site.	Stimulate 10–14 cm proximal to the active electrode over the radial side of the forearm.
Alternative Radial: Sensory (antidromic) (see Fig. A1.6)	Ring electrode over the metacarpal phalangeal joint of the thumb	Ring electrode over the interphalangeal joint of the thumb.	Place on the dorsum of the hand.	Stimulate 11 cm proximal to the active electrode, in the anatomical snuffbox.
Radial: Motor (see Fig. A1.7 and Video 4.7)	Place over the extensor indicis proprius on the dorsum of the forearm. Locate by extending the second digit. (A needle is sometimes used instead of a surface electrode.) Note that the amplitude of the CMAP cannot be compared if using a needle for the active electrode.	Place over the ulnar styloid.	Place between the active electrode and the stimulation site.	*Forearm:* Stimulate 4–6 cm proximal to the active electrode, over the ulna. *Elbow:* Stimulate in the groove between the biceps and the brachioradialis muscle. *Axilla:* Stimulate at the medial edge of the triceps (spiral groove) with the arm externally rotated and the forearm supinated.

Nerve	Active Electrode	Reference Electrode	Ground Electrode	Cathode
Lateral Antebrachial Cutaneous: Sensory (antidromic) (see Fig. A1.8 and Video 4.8)	Draw a line from the stimulation point to the radial styloid. Place the reference electrode 12cm distal to the cathode along this line.	Place the reference electrode 4cm distal to the active electrode.	Place between the active electrode and the stimulation site.	The cathode is placed at the elbow crease lateral to the biceps tendon.
Medial Antebrachial Cutaneous: Sensory (Video 4.9)	Halfway between the medial epicondyle and the ulnar styloid on the volar surface of the forearm.	If a bar electrode is not used, then the reference should be 4cm distal to the active electrode.	Place between the active electrode and the stimulation site.	In the antecubital fossa, proximal to the active electrode.
Musculocutaneous: Motor (see Fig. A1.9 and Video 4.10)	Place just distal to the midportion of the biceps muscle.	Place just proximal to the antecubital fossa, where the biceps tendon meets the muscle fibers.	Place over the deltoid muscle.	The cathode is placed above the upper clavicle and lateral to the sternocleidomastoid muscle. The anode is placed superiorly to the cathode (Erb's point).
Axillary: Motor (see Fig. A1.10 and Video 4.11)	Place on the middle of the deltoid muscle.	Place over the insertion of the deltoid on the lateral surface of the humerus.	Place between the active electrode and the stimulation site.	The cathode is placed lateral to where the sternocleidomastoid muscle meets the clavicle, just above the clavicle. The anode is placed superiorly and angled medially (Erb's point).
Fibular Motor (Peroneal)[a] (see Fig. A1.11 and Video 4.12)	Place on the anatomic center of the extensor digitorum brevis (EDB). Ask the patient to extend their toes and palpate for the muscle on the anterior lateral surface on the dorsum of the foot (usually located about 6cm from the lateral malleolus).	Place on the fifth toe.	Place between the active electrode and the stimulation site.	*Ankle:* Measure 8cm proximal to the EDB on the ankle, slightly lateral to the tibialis anterior tendon. *Fibula:* Stimulate below the head of the fibula anterior to the neck of the fibula. *Popliteal:* Measure at least 10cm proximal from the fibula, and stimulate in the lateral border of the popliteal fossa. Look for ankle dorsiflexion.
Sural: Sensory (see Fig. A1.12 and Video 4.13)	Place posterior to the lateral malleolus (about 2cm), and make sure it is parallel to the sole of the foot.	Place distal (at least 3cm) to the active electrode and parallel to the sole of the foot.	Place between the active electrode and the stimulation site.	Measure 14cm proximal from the active sure electrode near the midline of the gastrocnemius. Work your way laterally until an acceptable SNAP is achieved.
Tibial: Motor (see Fig. A1.13 and Video 4.14)	Place on the abductor hallucis muscle. Feel for the navicular bone of the foot and go 1 fingerbreadth toward the plantar surface of the foot and 1 fingerbreadth toward the great toe.	Place on the great toe's medial surface.	Place between the active electrode and the stimulation site.	Go slightly posterior to the medial malleolus and stimulate 10cm proximal to the active electrode. Stimulate in the popliteal fossa, slightly lateral to its midline. (Look for ankle plantar flexion with stimulation.)

Continued

TABLE 4.3 ■ **Nerve Conduction Studies Setup—Cont'd**

Nerve	Recording (Active) Electrode	Reference Electrode	Ground	Stimulation
Superficial Fibular (Peroneal): Sensory (see Fig. A1.14 and Video 4.15)	Place about 1 fingerbreadth medial to the lateral malleolus (between the tibialis anterior tendon and the lateral malleolus).	Place at least 3 cm distal to the active electrode.	Place on the anterior tibia between the active electrode and the stimulation site.	Stimulate 14 cm proximal to the active electrode along the anterior and the lateral surfaces of the leg.
Medial And Lateral Plantar Mixed: Sensory orthodromic (Video 4.16)	Over the tibial nerve posterior to the medial malleolus.	If a bar electrode is not used, then the reference should be 4 cm proximal to the active electrode.	Place between the active electrode and the stimulation site.	Stimulate 14 cm distal to the active electrode (approximating the course of the nerve). The medial plantar nerve is stimulated between the first and second metatarsals. The lateral plantar nerve is stimulated between the fourth and fifth metatarsals.
Sciatic (see Fig. A1.15)	Place on the EDB muscle (fibular component) or abductor hallucis muscle (tibial component).	Place on the small toe (fibular comp.) or the great toe (tibial comp.).	Place ground on the dorsum of the foot.	Stimulate using a needle in the middle of the gluteal fold.
Lateral Femoral Cutaneous: Antidromic (see Fig. A1.16)	Draw a line from the anterior superior iliac spine (ASIS) to the lateral border of the patella. Place the active electrode 16–18 cm distally along this line.	Place the reference electrode about 3 cm distal to the reference electrode along the same line connecting the ASIS and the lateral patella.	Place between the active electrode and the stimulation site.	Stimulate 1 cm medial to the ASIS. If using a cathode needle for stimulation, place a monopolar needle 1 cm medial to the ASIS, and place the anode several centimeters proximal.
H-Reflex (see Fig. A1.17 and Video 4.17)	Measure the distance between the popliteal crease and the medial malleolus. Place the active electrode halfway between the above-measured distance (over the medial gastrocnemius muscle).	Place on the Achilles tendon.	Place between the active electrode and the stimulation site.	Stimulate in the popliteal fossa, slightly lateral to the midline. Remember to turn the stimulator around with the cathode proximal to the anode. A stimulus just greater than that to evoke a minimal M response is applied to the posterior tibial nerve in the center of the popliteal crease.
F-Wave	Same setup used for motor nerve conduction of individual nerves.			Position the cathode proximal and use a supramaximal stimulus to the nerve using standard electrode placements.

[a]In many normal individuals, the EDB muscle may be atrophied. If low amplitude is obtained, it may be useful to place the active electrode over the tibialis anterior muscle and stimulate at the fibular head.

CAMP, Compound muscle action potential; SNAP, sensory nerve action potential.

- An increased duration (and smaller amplitude) on proximal stimulation could indicate a segmental demyelination in the segment being stimulated. In this situation (referred to as temporal dispersion), the area under the curve of the CMAP should not change. All of the axons are still contributing to the CMAP, but some are conducting much slower than others (see Fig. 4.7).

- A decrease of more than 20% amplitude with the proximal stimulation (compared to the distal amplitude) could indicate a conduction block across the segment. A conduction block occurs when an area of demyelination is so severe that saltatory conduction cannot occur. The action potential is *blocked* from propagating, and therefore those axons do not contribute to the amplitude of the CMAP. Remember, however, that this is a focal myelin problem, not an axonal problem, even though the amplitude is affected.

- With motor nerves, a distance of at least 10 cm between stimulation points should be used to decrease the likelihood of a measurement error significantly affecting the calculated conduction velocity. Because velocity = distance/time, a 1-cm error in measuring over a 5-cm distance will result in a 20% error in distance and will significantly affect the calculated conduction velocity. If the distance is 10 cm, a 1-cm error results in only a 10% error in distance. Generally, due to skin elasticity and other factors, a measurement will be accurate to within about 1 cm. In obese patients, there may be a decreased ability to accurately measure the length of the nerve segment.

- You can estimate the amount of axonal loss in an acute peripheral nerve lesion if you compare the amplitude of the CMAP on the unaffected side. For example, if the amplitude of a median CMAP is 10 mV on the nonaffected side and 5 mV on the affected side, you can estimate that approximately 50% of the axons have been lost.

- When stimulating the ulnar nerve, the elbow should be bent to 70 to 90 degrees. If the elbow is held straight, the calculated conduction velocity will be falsely decreased. This is because the nerve is slack in the extended position and the distance is falsely decreased. If the numerator (distance) in the equation velocity = distance/time is decreased, the velocity will be decreased. In addition, if both elbows are not held in the same position, there will be a false side-to-side velocity difference.

Table 4.3 describes the proper placement of electrodes for the most commonly used motor and sensory studies (see Appendix 1 for illustrations). For the normal values of most peripheral nerve studies, see Chapter 25, Tables of Normals.

Reference

1. American Association of Neuromuscular & Electrodiagnostic Medicine (AANEM). Proper performance and interpretation of electrodiagnostic studies. *Muscle Nerve*. 2006;33:436–439.

CHAPTER 5

Electromyography

Lyn D. Weiss ■ Jay M. Weiss

Electromyographic (EMG) testing involves evaluation of the electrical activity of a muscle and is one of the fundamental parts of the electrodiagnostic medical consultation. It is both an art and a science. It requires a thorough knowledge of the anatomy of the muscles being tested, the machine settings, and the neurophysiology behind the testing.

The EMG portion of the test involves putting a very thin needle into a muscle and assessing the electrical activity of the muscle. The electromyographer must be cognizant that the test is inherently uncomfortable. It is important to obtain the confidence and cooperation of the patient. Most patients are more comfortable when time is taken to explain the reasons for the testing and what information can be gained from the testing. It is a fallacy that the test is comfortable, and any attempt to convince a patient that it is comfortable is certain to fail. Some things that can be done to allay the patient's fears are performing the study in a quiet room, speaking in a confident and calming manner, playing music of the patient's choice, and keeping the room temperature comfortable.

Muscle Physiology

EMG assesses skeletal or voluntary muscle (rather than smooth or cardiac muscle). The muscle fibers that account for the strength of a contraction are extrafusal fibers (as opposed to intrafusal fibers of the muscle spindle). The extrafusal fibers are relaxed at rest with an intracellular resting potential of approximately −80 mV (similar to nerve fibers). The sarcolemma is a plasma membrane surrounding a muscle fiber. The action potential from a motor nerve fiber will synapse at the neuromuscular junction (NMJ) and then propagate along the sarcolemma. The sarcolemma has extensions into the muscle fibers called T tubules. The depolarization of the T tubules causes release of calcium from the sarcoplasmic reticulum. The calcium release results in changes in the actin and myosin. This shortens the actin–myosin functional unit, resulting in muscle contraction. EMG measures the electrical excitation of the muscle fibers.

Motor Units

Muscles contract and produce movement through the orderly recruitment of motor units. A *motor unit* (MU) is defined as one anterior horn cell, its axon, and all the muscle fibers innervated by that anterior horn cell (the cell including the axon is called a motor neuron). An MU is the fundamental structure that is assessed in electromyography. The *MU architecture* refers to its size, distribution, and endplate area. When a person starts to contract a muscle, the first MUs to fire are usually the smallest. These are the Type I MUs. As the contraction increases, there is an orderly recruitment of larger MUs (which have a higher threshold). They begin to fire and add to the force of the contraction.

Before You Begin

Most students of electrodiagnostic medicine are a little intimidated by the needle part of the test. Sometimes, practicing with an orange can help you get the feel of the needle and how to position it. The *feel* of transitioning the needle between the rind and the pulp of an orange is similar to piercing the muscle after inserting the needle through the skin. In keeping with the first tenet of medicine, "first do no harm," it is important to know where to place the needle and why you are testing a certain muscle so as not to subject the patient to unnecessary needle testing. A good working knowledge of muscle anatomy is an essential tool for placing the needle in the appropriate muscle.

Electrodes

Just as with nerve conduction studies, you need a ground, a reference, and a recording electrode. The needle is the *recording electrode*; the reference may be separate or part of the needle itself. If the reference is separate, it should be placed over the same muscle that is being tested by the needle. The ground can be placed anywhere on the extremity being tested.

Universal precautions must always be practiced during the needle portion of the test. This is to protect you as well as the patient. Universal precautions include use of gloves, proper needle disposal, and use of a one-handed technique for needle recapping. This can be done by securing the needle cover to the preamplifier and using one hand to place the needle back in the cover between muscle testing (Fig. 5.1).

TYPES OF NEEDLE ELECTRODES

Monopolar Needle

Monopolar needles are made of stainless steel and have a fine point insulated except at the distal 0.2 to 0.4 mm segment (Fig. 5.2). They require a surface electrode placed over the same muscle as a reference. A separate surface electrode placed on the skin serves as a ground. A monopolar needle records the voltage changes between the tip of the electrode and the reference. The amplitude of the waveform recorded from a monopolar needle is usually larger than one recorded from a concentric needle. The concentric needle records from a 180-degree field, whereas the monopolar records from a full 360-degree field around the needle. When a muscle contracts, potentials are recorded by both the recording and reference electrodes. Through the process of differential amplification, the common signals are rejected. A monopolar needle also has a smaller diameter and a Teflon or similar coating. This makes the monopolar less uncomfortable than a concentric needle. This, combined with its cost advantage over the concentric, has led to its widespread clinical use.

Standard or Concentric Needle

A concentric needle is a stainless steel cannula similar to a hypodermic needle with a wire in the center of the shaft (Fig. 5.3). The pointed tip of the needle has an oval shape. While the wire is bare at the tip, the shaft can conduct electrical activity along its entire length. The needle, when near a source of electrical activity, registers the potential difference between the wire and the shaft. It is important to remember that the exposed recording electrode is on the beveled portion of the cannula and thus is picking up from one direction (180 degrees rather than 360 degrees as in a monopolar needle). A separate surface electrode serves as the ground. Some electromyographers think that the concentric electrode is less *noisy* than the monopolar electrode, providing a clearer signal.

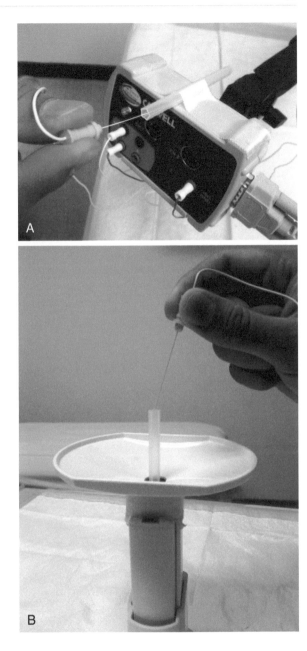

Fig. 5.1   Needle recapping.

Bipolar Concentric Needle

The cannula of the bipolar needle contains two fine stainless steel or platinum wires (Fig. 5.4). This electrode is larger in diameter than the standard coaxial concentric needle. It registers the potential electrical difference between the two inside wires while the cannula serves as the ground. The bipolar needle detects potentials from a much smaller area than the standard coaxial concentric needle. This needle is also slightly more uncomfortable than a monopolar needle because of its increased diameter. This electrode is used primarily for research, not in routine clinical studies.

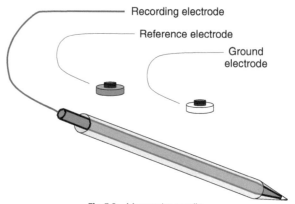

Fig. 5.2 Monopolar needle.

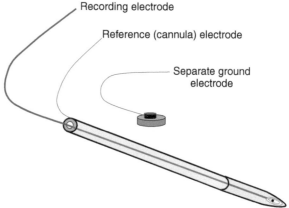

Fig. 5.3 Concentric needle.

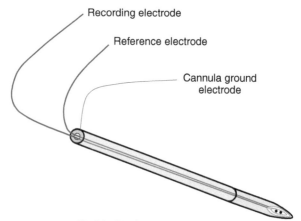

Fig. 5.4 Bipolar concentric needle.

Single-Fiber Needle

Single-fiber needles may contain two or more wires exposed along the shaft serving as the leading edge to record from individual muscle fibers rather than MUs. These electrodes are used to assess NMJ transmission and fiber density, topics that are beyond the scope of this text.

Planning the Examination

It is important to plan out which muscles you will test before you begin. This plan may change as you proceed, depending on the results of the muscles being tested. If you think the patient will be able to tolerate only a limited number of muscles, start with the ones that will contribute the most to your diagnosis. The test is uncomfortable, and many people are afraid of needles. Therefore, try to test as few muscles as possible without sacrificing the quality of the examination.

Starting the Test

The EMG examination can be divided into four components:
- insertional activity,
- examination of the muscle at rest,
- analysis of the MU, and
- recruitment.

Prior to evaluating insertional activity and examination of the muscle at rest, it is important to make sure that the low-frequency filter is set at 10 to 30 Hz, the high-frequency filter is set at 10,000 to 20,000 Hz (10 to 20 kHz), the amplifier sensitivity is set at 50 to 100 microvolts (μV) per division, and the sweep speed is typically set at 10 msec per division. Always cleanse the skin with alcohol thoroughly before inserting the needle. The needle should be inserted into the muscle quickly and deliberately. Tensing the skin will allow quicker needle insertion and less discomfort to the patient.

For the first two components of the examination, insertional activity and examination of the resting muscle, the needle electrode is directed through the muscle in four quadrants. Each of these quadrants can be examined at three or four different depths, allowing 12 to 16 discrete areas of muscle to be examined electrically. The EMG has been likened to an *electrical biopsy*; and, as with any biopsy, the more areas examined, the less chance of false negatives.

INSERTIONAL ACTIVITY

Healthy muscle at rest is electrically silent as soon as needle movement stops (as long as the end-plate region is avoided). During this portion of the examination, the muscle being tested should be at rest. The best way to electrically silence the muscle (if the patient cannot relax it) is to tell the patient to contract the antagonist muscle (or reposition the extremity so the muscle is relaxed). For example, if you put a needle in the biceps muscle and the patient's elbow is bent, MUs in the biceps muscle are probably firing. Telling the patient to straighten the elbow will activate MUs in the triceps muscle (and inactivate MUs in the biceps muscle). Because it is extremely difficult to activate both the agonist and antagonist muscles at the same time, the agonist muscle usually will relax. (Remember that the biceps muscle is also a supinator. Therefore, pronating the arm is important to put the biceps muscle at rest. Here again, a working knowledge of where muscles are located, what they do, and which nerves innervate them is essential.)

If the needle is properly placed in the muscle you are testing, you will hear and see brief electrical activity associated with the needle movement. This is called *insertional activity*. The sound associated with this needle movement has been described as *crisp* and is temporally related to the high-frequency positive and negative spikes that are easily visualized on the monitor. If the patient can tolerate it, this should be done in four different quadrants and at four different depths. To reposition the needle, pull it back carefully to the plane where the muscle and fascia transition (with practice, you will soon be able to *feel* when you leave the muscle) and then insert the needle at a new angle. Try not to pull back too far, or you will pull the needle all the way out and have to restick the needle into the patient.

Normal insertional activity typically lasts only a few hundred milliseconds, just barely longer than the needle movement itself. It is thought to be generated by the needle tip physically depolarizing the muscle fibers as it pierces and/or displaces them.

Decreased insertional activity occurs when the needle is inserted into an *atrophied* muscle. The sensation of inserting the needle has been described as putting a needle into sand. Remember that the initial sound and EMG recording of needle insertion into muscle is actually the muscle fiber being injured by needle movement. With muscle atrophy, there will be decreased response to needle insertion, because there is less muscle tissue. Caution should be used in interpretation, especially without clinically visible muscle wasting, to make sure that the needle is indeed in muscle and not in other tissue, such as adipose or connective tissue.

Increased insertional activity may occur when there is muscle pathology and is evidenced by the presence of positive sharp waves (PSWs) and/or *fibrillation potentials* (fibs) that are apparent only on insertion and *do not persist*. Increased insertional activity may precede actual denervation. On insertion, any electrical activity that lasts longer than 300 msec is considered increased. These determinations require a subjective assessment based on the experience of the electromyographer (Fig. 5.5).

EXAMINATION OF THE MUSCLE AT REST

Once the needle is inserted into the muscle, pause several seconds to assess for spontaneous activity. Normal muscles should be electrically silent after needle insertion. For this portion of the test, the muscle should be at rest.

Spontaneous Activity

Spontaneous activity is typically abnormal and occurs in the presence of pathology. Normal muscle has a resting membrane potential of $-80\,mV$ relative to the extracellular fluids. After injury or denervation, the membrane potential becomes more positive due to an influx of Na^+ into the

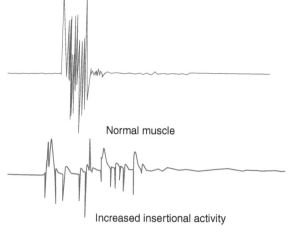

Normal muscle

Increased insertional activity

Fig. 5.5 *(Top)* Normal insertional activity. *(Bottom)* Increased insertional activity.

damaged cell membrane. The muscle cell tends to become less negative and therefore closer to the potential needed for the generation of spontaneous action potentials. This occurs when the cell resting membrane potential reaches −60 mV.

The term *denervation potentials* is a misnomer and should not be used to describe spontaneous activity. *Spontaneous activity* is a more appropriate term. Irritation can be brought about by many factors other than nerve injury (such as metabolic or inflammatory muscle disease, local muscle trauma, or excessive needle probing of the muscle). Either the muscle or the nerve may generate spontaneous activity (Table 5.1).

PSWs, fibrillations, fasciculations, complex repetitive discharges (CRDs), and *myotonic discharges* are examples of abnormal spontaneous potentials that are generated at the level of the muscle fiber. Abnormal findings due to a dysfunction of the neural input to the muscle can lead to the development of *myokymic* discharges as well as *cramps, neuromyotonic discharges, tremors, multiples*, and *fasciculations*. The more common types of spontaneous activity are described below. Because of their small amplitude, the gain on the EMG machine must be set at 50 to 100 µV in order for the potentials to be visualized.

PSWs are muscle fiber action potentials that can be recorded from a muscle with impaired muscle innervation or from an injured portion of a muscle. PSWs consist of a primary positive (downward) deflection from the baseline (positive wave) followed by a return to the baseline. These waves are either monophasic or biphasic in morphology (Fig. 5.6). They tend to fire regularly at a rate of 0.5 to 15 Hz. Amplitudes tend to vary between 20 and 1000 µV. PSWs sound like dull thuds and tend to appear earlier than fibs after a muscle is deprived of its nerve supply.

TABLE 5.1 ■ Spontaneous Activity Generated by Muscle or Nerve

Spontaneous Activity Generated by the Muscle
Fibrillation potentials (fibs)
Positive sharp waves (PSWs)
Myotonic discharges
Complex repetitive discharges (CRDs)
Fasciculations[a]

Spontaneous Activity Generated by the Nerve
Myokymic discharges
Cramps
Neuromyotonic discharges
Tremors
Multiples
Fasciculations[a]

[a]Fasciculations can be considered muscle or nerve generated.

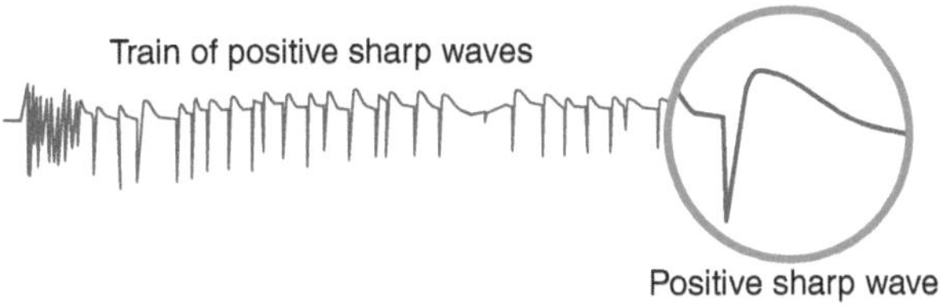

Train of positive sharp waves

Fig. 5.6 Positive sharp wave.

Positive sharp wave

Fibs are the spontaneous action potentials of single muscle fibers that are firing autonomously. These can occur in the presence of impaired innervation. This process repeats on a time interval dependent upon the repolarization-to-threshold turnaround time. These potentials usually fire in a regular pattern at rates of 0.5 to 15 Hz. The fibs are usually triphasic in morphology and range from 20 to 1000 µV in size (Fig. 5.7). They sound like raindrops hitting a tin roof. Fibs and PSWs may be recorded in both neurogenic and myopathic disease states, and when seen on EMG, they signify essentially the same thing: spontaneous discharge of the muscle fibers, most often due to impaired innervation of the muscle being tested (Table 5.2). In fact, some authors refer to both PSWs and fibs as fibs, and do not distinguish one from the other. They regard the different appearances as a function of the location of the needle electrode.

Spontaneous fibs and PSWs are usually reported on a scale from 0 to 4. Zero means that no fibs or PSWs are present. The rest of the grading is subjective. As a general rule, if one PSW or fib is seen per screen (using a sweep of 10 msec per division), the score is +1. In this situation, the fibs or PSWs may not be present in every area of the muscle. If spontaneous potentials are present in more than one area of the muscle or are more numerous, the score is +2. If fibs and PSWs essentially fill the screen, they are graded as +4.

Fibs and PSWs usually indicate a process of acute or ongoing impaired innervation. These spontaneous potentials, however, may not be seen on EMG testing until 2 weeks or more after an injury. See Chapter 6, Injuries to Peripheral Nerves, for further details on timing of EMG findings after nerve injury.

CRDs are groups of spontaneously firing action potentials. The etiology of the CRD is a local muscular *arrhythmia* with an affected area of muscle electrically stimulating adjacent muscle

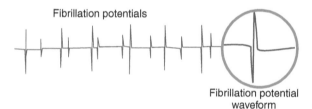

Fibrillation potentials

Fibrillation potential waveform

Fig. 5.7 Fibrillation.

TABLE 5.2 ■ Conditions Associated With Positive Sharp Waves and Fibrillation Potentials

Chronic Muscle Disorders
- Inflammatory myopathies
- Inclusion body myositis
- Congenital myopathies
- Rhabdomyolysis
- Muscle trauma
- Trichinosis

Neurogenic Disorders
- Radiculopathy
- Axonal peripheral neuropathy
- Plexopathies
- Entrapment neuropathies
- Motor neuron disease
- Mononeuritis

fibers and therefore perpetuating the rhythm. CRDs appear as runs of simple or complex spike patterns that repeat in a regular pattern. They have a frequency of between 10 and 100 Hz. The amplitudes of the responses are between 50 and 500 μV. These potentials start and stop abruptly (Fig. 5.8). They have a uniform frequency and sound like motorboats that misfire occasionally. These potentials are seen in both neurogenic and myopathic disorders (Table 5.3). They tend to be seen in more long-standing disorders and are suggestive that the injury is greater than 6 months old.

Myotonic discharges are the action potentials of muscle fibers firing in prolonged fashions after activation and are noted on needle insertion. Clinically this state is seen as delayed relaxation of a muscle after a forceful contraction. This may also be seen after striking a muscle belly with a reflex hammer, as in percussion myotonia. Myotonic discharges have two potential forms. The wave may have either PSW morphology or a pattern of biphasic or triphasic potentials. These potentials tend to fire at variable rates with waxing and waning appearances. The frequency varies between 20 and 100 Hz (Fig. 5.9). This variation in frequency gives the discharge its characteristic *dive-bomber* sound. Myotonic discharges may be found in the following conditions: myotonic dystrophy, myotonia congenita, paramyotonia, hyperkalemic periodic paralysis, polymyositis, acid maltase deficiency, and chronic radiculopathy and neuropathies.

Myokymic discharges are groups of spontaneous MU potentials that have regular firing patterns and rhythms. They are seen in two forms. In the continuous form, they are seen as single or paired discharges of MU potentials that fire at rates from 5 to 10 Hz. In the discontinuous form,

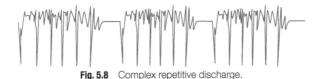

Fig. 5.8   Complex repetitive discharge.

Fig. 5.9   Myotonic discharges. Note waxing and waning in frequency and amplitude.

TABLE 5.3 ■ **Conditions Associated With Complex Repetitive Discharges**

Chronic Muscle Disorders
1. Myopathies
2. Polymyositis
3. Limb-girdle dystrophy
4. Myxedema
5. Schwartz–Jampel syndrome

Neurogenic Disorders
1. Chronic neuropathies
2. Poliomyelitis
3. Spinal muscular atrophy
4. Motor neuron disease
5. Hereditary neuropathies

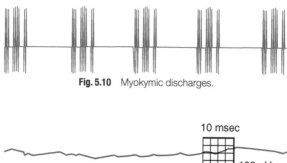

Fig. 5.10   Myokymic discharges.

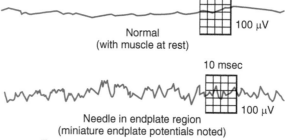

Fig. 5.11   Miniature endplate potentials (MEPPs).

they are seen as bursts of motor potentials that repeat at rates from 0.1 to 10 Hz. This form of the myokymic response sounds like soldiers marching (Fig. 5.10). Myokymic responses may be seen in facial muscles in Bell's palsy, multiple sclerosis, and polyradiculopathy. They are also seen in limb muscles in chronic nerve lesions and in radiation plexopathy. The term *myokymia* is used clinically to describe a *wormlike* quivering of the muscle. However, this clinical finding is usually associated with neuromyotonic rather than myokymic discharges on EMG.

Endplate Region

Healthy muscle should have no *spontaneous activity* unless the needle is in the endplate region of a muscle fiber (where the nerve enters the muscle). If the needle is in the endplate region, it should be repositioned, because you are not likely to ascertain anything about a muscle from this location and it can be quite painful for the patient. There are three things to look for that may tell you the needle is in the endplate region:

1. miniature endplate potentials (MEPPs), which give a characteristic seashell sound,
2. *endplate spikes*, and
3. *pain*. (The patient may feel a dull ache or increased pain relative to other positions.)

MEPPs are believed to represent the spontaneous release of acetylcholine (ACh) at the pre-synaptic terminal. When ACh attaches to the receptors, there is subsequent activation of the sodium and potassium channels of the muscle, which in turn creates a small current.

Endplate spikes are believed to be single muscle-fiber depolarizations. A needle may cause sufficient irritation to the presynaptic nerve terminal to release a large amount of ACh. This may subsequently produce a threshold adequate for depolarization.

Endplate spikes and MEPPs do not necessarily have to be found together. *MEPPs* are of short duration (1 to 2 msec), fire with irregular activity every few seconds or so, are small (10 to 20 μV), and have monophasic negative (upward) waveforms (Fig. 5.11). *Endplate spikes* are typically biphasic with initial negative deflections, are of intermediate amplitude (about 100 to 200 μV), and have longer durations than MEPPs (3 to 5 msec). Like MEPPs, they fire irregularly. The endplates should be avoided because of patient discomfort and possible interpretation errors. (Positive waves in the endplate do not indicate denervation, can be mistaken for fibs or PSWs, and are normal findings.) To move away from the endplate, advance the needle slightly and firmly. Now the muscle should be electrically quiet, and the patient should be more comfortable.

ANALYZING THE MOTOR UNIT ACTION POTENTIAL

Once the muscle has been assessed for insertional activity and activity at rest, the MU itself should be analyzed. During this portion of the needle test, the patient is asked to *minimally* contract the muscle. Too often, electromyographers tell the patient to maximally contract the muscle. If the muscle is fully contracted, it is almost impossible to isolate and therefore analyze individual MUs.

When analyzing MUs, the sweep speed should be set at 10 msec per division and the gain should be 500 to 1000 mV per division. Most assessments of MU morphology can be made more accurately by freezing the screen or by using a trigger and delay line. Trigger and delay lines are obtained on most EMG machines by pressing a button. This is necessary for a detailed analysis of MUs. The trigger is set to record a tracing when a certain amplitude threshold is reached. When a potential exceeds the trigger threshold, that potential is displayed on the screen. That potential remains on the screen until the next potential reaches threshold. Then the new potential replaces the previous potential. This allows the electromyographer to *freeze* a motor unit action potential (MUAP) above a certain amplitude and analyze it.

At low levels of contraction (when few MUs are firing), slight movements of the needle can *tune in* the desired potential. At this point, the same potential will be constantly replaced in the same location on the screen. The delay line determines the position of the potential on the screen. Thus the placement of the delay line determines how much time before and after the potential being examined is being displayed. The *strobe* effect of potentials being locked into the same position allows detailed analysis of all components of MU morphology including amplitude, duration, and number of phases as well as stability. Subtle changes can become apparent. ⅰ

In addition, satellite potentials, separated from the main MUAP by an isoelectric interval, fire in a time-locked relationship to the main action potential. These potentials usually follow, but they may precede the main action potential in the same location and therefore become apparent. These will likely be evident only in this manner because, without a trigger and delay function, they may appear as different MUs. The trigger and delay function is an extremely valuable tool in performing MU analysis.

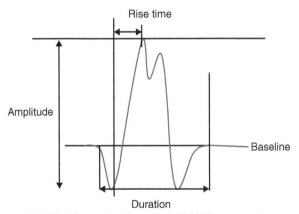

Fig. 5.12 Motor unit action potential (MUAP) components.

Components of the Motor Unit

Analysis of the MU morphology should include an assessment of the following parameters: (1) amplitude, (2) rise time, (3) duration, (4) phases, and (5) stability. Fig. 5.12 depicts the various components of the MUAP morphology.

Amplitude. In a healthy motor neuron, all of the muscle fibers discharge in near synchrony. Muscle fibers located near the tip of the electrode make the greatest contribution to the amplitude of the MU potential. Their contribution to the amplitude decreases significantly as the distance from the needle tip increases. Therefore the *same* MU can give rise to potentials of *different* amplitude and appearance at different recording sites.

MUAP amplitude is measured from the most positive to the most negative peak, and it reflects fiber density. Amplitude of the MUs may be *normal, increased,* or *decreased.* With a concentric needle, amplitude ranges from several hundred microvolts to a few millivolts. Amplitudes are larger with a monopolar needle (normally 1 to 7 mV) because the monopolar needle picks up electrical activity from a full 360-degree field around the needle. Increased amplitude of MUs can be noted with reinnervation, as is seen with neuropathic injuries after a period of months. Decreased amplitude may be seen in myopathies. Amplitude increases (1) as the needle approximates the MU, (2) as you increase the number of muscle fibers of the MU, (3) with increasing diameter of the muscle fibers (muscle fiber hypertrophy), and (4) with more synchronous firing of the muscle fibers.

Rise Time. Rise time is defined as the time lag from the initial positive deflection to the subsequent negative upward peak. This helps estimate the distance between the recording tip and discharging MU. The more vertical the waveform, the shorter (quicker) the rise time. A distant MU has a longer rise time because the resistance and capacitance of the intervening tissue act as high-frequency filters. A unit accepted for qualitative measurement should produce a sharp sound, while a distant unit will produce a dull sound indicating the need to reposition the needle electrode closer to the source. An acceptable rise time is 0.5 msec or less.

Duration. Duration is measured from the initial departure from baseline to the final return to the baseline. Normal duration is about 11 msec. It indicates the degree of synchrony of firing among all individual muscle fibers with variable lengths, conduction velocities, and membrane excitabilities. A slight shift in the needle position influences the duration much less than the amplitude.

When all the fibers of an MU fire in relative synchrony, the duration will be short. If there is asynchrony of firing (e.g., with reinnervation), the duration will be longer. Increased duration is seen in neuropathic processes, while decreased duration is seen in myopathic disorders. Duration is decreased in myopathies because fewer muscle fibers contribute to the MU.

Phases. A phase is the portion of the waveform between the successive crossings of the baseline. The number of phases, which is determined by counting negative and positive peaks, equals the number of times the baseline is crossed plus one. Normally, MU potentials have four or fewer phases. Polyphasic MUs (more than four phases) suggest desynchronized discharge or drop-off of individual fibers. Normal muscles may have up to 15% polyphasic MUAPs when using a concentric needle and up to 30% polyphasic MUAPs when using a monopolar needle. If an increased percentage of the MUs consists of five or more phases, the MUs of that muscle are considered polyphasic. MU duration is a better measure of pathology than polyphasicity.

Stability. The morphology of an MU should be stable in normal MUAPs. Unstable MUAP morphology (changes in amplitude or number of phases) occurs in primary disorders of the NMJ or disorders associated with new or immature NMJs (reinnervation). The trigger and delay function (which places any MU that exceeds a selected amplitude in the same spot on the screen so that it can be analyzed) may be helpful.

RECRUITMENT

Recruitment is an often misunderstood and misused term. Recruitment refers to the *orderly addition of MUs* so as to *increase the force of a contraction.* A contraction becomes stronger in two ways: the firing MUs *increase their rate of firing* and *additional MUs commence firing.*

The machine settings for evaluating recruitment should be a sweep of 10 msec per division and a gain of 500 to 1000 mV per division. Recruitment analysis should begin with the patient being told to think about contracting the muscle being analyzed. Observe for the firing of a single MUAP. It usually begins to fire at 2 to 3 Hz in an *irregular* pattern.

Normally the MU will fire in a *regular* pattern at about 5 Hz. At around 10 Hz, another MUAP will be recruited to fire. The new MU will initially fire at about 5 Hz. The normal firing rate of most MUs, before additional units are recruited, is 10 Hz. To calculate the firing rate of the MU, note how many times an MU with an identical morphology repeats across a screen set at 100 msec per screen (sweep speed of 10 msec per division). Multiply that number by 10 to get the MU firing per 1000 msec or 1 s. Remember that Hz indicates cycles per second. In a neuropathic process, some MUs will be unavailable to fire (Fig. 5.13). An MU that is able to fire will try to "make up for" the inability of other units to fire by firing at a higher frequency. Therefore the MU will have an increased firing frequency before another MU is recruited, which is referred to as *decreased recruitment.* In decreased recruitment, there are fewer MUs firing at a higher frequency. *Recruitment ratio* is another term used to describe the firing rate of an MU. This ratio is the rate of firing of the most rapidly firing MU (in Hz) divided by the number of units firing. A recruitment ratio of over 8 is considered abnormal and suggests a neurogenic process.

Neuropathic recruitment, also called *neurogenic recruitment,* can be seen in neuropathies, radiculopathies, motor neuron disease, and trauma. Few MUs fire at an increased rate or firing frequency (Fig. 5.13). The firing rates of these MUAPs are greater than 20 Hz (20 cycles per second) and may increase to 30 Hz or more. Pathologic states can tell us much about physiology. In severe neuropathic lesions, when there are few functional MUs, we can see MUs firing at 30 Hz before a second MU in that area is recruited. This indicates that weakness is not due to pain or poor effort but to physiologic factors. Functional MUs are simply not available. If only a few MUs are firing

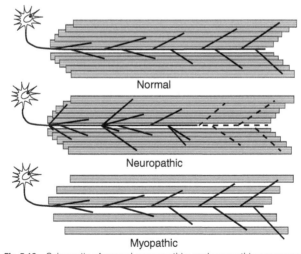

Fig. 5.13 Schematic of normal, neuropathic, and myopathic processes.

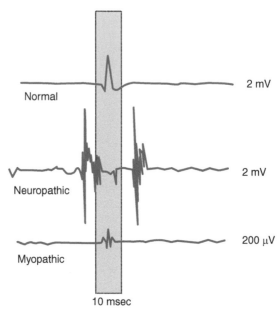

Normal

2 mV

Neuropathic

2 mV

Myopathic

200 µV

10 msec

Fig. 5.14 Normal, neuropathic, and myopathic recruitments.

but they are firing at a normal rate, recruitment is normal. The decreased activation of the muscle may be due to either decreased effort or to a central nervous system lesion.

The terms *increased recruitment* and *early recruitment* are sometimes used to describe a myopathic process. In myopathic recruitment, a large number of MUs are *recruited* for a minimal contraction. In myopathies, the individual muscle fiber contribution to each MU is reduced (see Fig. 5.13). Because myopathic fibers cannot increase their force outputs, they quickly recruit additional MUs to increase the force of a contraction. In this situation, one MU will fire at only about 5 Hz before the next MU is recruited. If referring to the recruitment ratio, there will be a decreased rate of firing (numerator) per number of MUs recruited (denominator). Recruitment ratios below 3 suggest a myopathic process.

Myopathic MUAPs tend to have an *early* recruitment of *short*-duration, *low*-amplitude MUAPs firing at increased rates (Fig. 5.14). In a myopathy, it is difficult to obtain only one or two MUs per screen at minimal contraction. Polyphasicity and spontaneous potentials can be seen in myopathies (as in neuropathies). Because these MUs have low amplitude, analysis cannot be done adequately with a trigger and delay or capture function but must be done with a constant sweep.

In EMG evaluation of MUAP recruitment, it is important to realize that we are primarily evaluating Type I MUs because they recruit first. By the time the Type II fibers recruit, the baseline will be obscured by Type I potentials. This is problematic in those myopathies that involve predominately Type II fibers, such as steroid myopathies, because only the Type I fibers are evaluated. In steroid myopathies, even though the patient has a myopathy clinically and on biopsy, the needle EMG may be normal.

Summary

EMG evaluation requires patience and effort on the parts of both the electromyographer and the patient. The amount of information obtained from the test is dependent upon appropriate planning and selection of the muscles as well as experience in waveform recognition. Table 5.4 reviews the common muscles tested during the needle portion of the examination and the muscle's innervation, location, and needle placement. This table will help you plan which muscles to test and how to ensure proper needle placement. This is a relatively comprehensive list, and it is rare that most (or even many) of these muscles will be necessary in an individual study. The choice of muscles to be examined should be dictated by the clinical circumstances.

Many muscles are very close together (e.g., in the forearm). Due to individual differences in size (and, less often, to differences in anatomy) and to depth of needle insertion, the needle may not always be in the desired muscle. A test maneuver may be necessary to confirm needle placement. Activate the muscle. If the needle is in the muscle being activated, large, crisp MUs will be seen and heard. Table 5.5 compares some of the more common potentials seen on needle testing and when they might be noted.

TABLE 5.4 ■ Common Muscles—Innervation, Location, and Needle Placement (See Video 5.1)

Muscle	Nerve	Cord	Division	Trunk	C4	C5	C6	C7	C8
Sternocleidomastoid (see Fig. A2.1)	Spinal accessory nerve	CN XI, C2, C3							
Trapezius (see Fig. A2.2)	Spinal accessory nerve	CN XI, C3			C4				
Rhomboid major (see Fig. A2.3)	Dorsal scapular nerve	N/A	N/A	Upper trunk		C5			
Rhomboid minor (see Fig. A2.3)	Dorsal scapular nerve	N/A	N/A	Upper trunk		C5			
Levator scapulae (see Fig. A2.4)	Dorsal scapular nerve	N/A	N/A	Upper trunk	C3, C4	C5			
Supraspinatus (see Fig. A2.5)	Suprascapular nerve	N/A	N/A	Upper trunk		C5	C6		
Infraspinatus (see Fig. A2.6)	Suprascapular nerve	N/A	N/A	Upper trunk		C5	C6		
Teres major (see Fig. A2.7)	Lower subscapular nerve	Posterior cord	Posterior division	Upper trunk		C5	C6	C7	
Deltoid (see Fig. A2.8 and Video 5.2)	Circumflex (axillary) nerve	Posterior cord	Posterior division	Upper trunk		C5	C6		
Teres minor (see Fig. A2.9)	Circumflex (axillary) nerve	Posterior cord	Posterior division	Upper trunk		C5	C6		
Coracobrachialis (see Fig. A2.10)	Musculocutaneous nerve	Lateral cord	Anterior division	Upper and middle trunk		C5	C6	C7	
Biceps brachii (see Fig. A2.11 and Video 5.3)	Musculocutaneous nerve	Lateral cord	Anterior division	Upper trunk		C5	C6		
Brachialis (see Fig. A2.12)	Musculocutaneous nerve	Lateral cord	Anterior division	Upper trunk		C5	C6		
Latissimus dorsi (see Fig. A2.13)	Thoracodorsal nerve	Posterior cord	Posterior division	Upper, middle, and lower trunk			C6	C7	C8

T1	Needle Insertion	Origin	Insertion	Action
	At the midpoint between the mastoid process and the sternal origin. Enter the muscle obliquely and direct the needle parallel to the muscle fibers.	The sternal head arises from the upper part of the manubrium sterni. The clavicular head arises from the medial third of the clavicle.	The lateral surface of the mastoid process	Rotates the head
	At the angle of the neck and shoulder or midway between the spine of the scapula and the spinous processes at the same level	External occipital protuberance, superior nuchal line, ligamentum nuchae, spines of C7–T12	Spine of the scapula, acromion, lateral third of the clavicle	Adducts, rotates, elevates, and depresses scapula
	At the midpoint of the medial scapular border, midway between the scapular spine and the inferior angle	Spines of T2–T5	Medial border of scapula	Adducts the scapula
	At the point just medial to the medial border of the scapular spine	Spines of C7–T1	Root of the spine of the scapula	Adducts the scapula
	At the posteromedial border of the scapula, between the superior angle and the spine of the scapula	The transverse processes of the upper four cervical vertebrae	The posteromedial border of the scapula, between the superior angle and the spine of the scapula	Elevates the scapula
	At the supraspinous fossa just above the spine of the scapula	Supraspinous fossa of the scapula	Superior facet of the greater tubercle of the humerus	Abducts the arm
	At the midpoint of the infraspinous fossa	Infraspinous fossa	Middle facet of the greater tubercle of the humerus	Rotates the arm laterally
	Along the lateral lower border of the scapula (lateral and rostral to the inferior angle)	Dorsal surface of the inferior angle of the scapula	Medial lip of the intertubercular groove of the humerus	Adducts and rotates the arm medially
	5 cm beneath the lateral border of the acromion	Lateral third of the clavicle, acromion, and spine of the scapula	Deltoid tuberosity of the humerus	Abducts, adducts, flexes, extends, and rotates the arm medially
	Immediately lateral to the middle third of the lateral border of the scapula	Upper portion of lateral border of the scapula	Lower facet of the greater tubercle of the humerus	Rotates the arm laterally
	5–9 cm distal to the coracoid process along the volar aspect of the arm	Coracoid process	Middle third of the medial surface of the humerus	Flexes and adducts the arm
	At the mid arm anteriorly, into the bulk of the muscle	Long head, supraglenoid tubercle; short head, coracoid process	Radial tuberosity of the radius	Flexes and supinates the forearm; assists in flexion of the arm at the shoulder
	5 cm proximal to the elbow crease just lateral to and under the biceps	Lower anterior surface of the humerus	Coronoid process of the ulna and the ulnar tuberosity	Flexes the forearm at the elbow
	Along the posterior axillary fold directly lateral to the inferior angle of the scapula	Spines of T7–T12 thoracolumbar fascia, iliac crest, 9th to 12th ribs	Floor of the bicipital groove of the humerus	Adducts, extends, and medially rotates the arm

Continued

TABLE 5.4 ■ Common Muscles—Innervation, Location, and Needle Placement (See Video 5.1)—Cont'd

Muscle	Nerve	Cord	Division	Trunk	C4	C5	C6	C7	C8
Serratus anterior (see Fig. A2.14)	Long thoracic nerve	Anterior rami				C5	C6	C7	
Triceps (see Fig. A2.15 and Video 5.4)	Radial nerve	Posterior cord	Posterior division	Upper, middle, and lower trunk			C6	C7	C8
Anconeus (see Fig. A2.16)	Radial nerve	Posterior cord	Posterior division	Upper, middle, and lower trunk			C6	C7	C8
Brachioradialis (see Fig. A2.17 and Video 5.5)	Radial nerve	Posterior cord	Posterior division	Upper trunk		C5	C6		
Extensor carpi radialis (see Fig. A2.18)	Radial nerve	Posterior cord	Posterior division	Upper and middle trunk			C6	C7	
Supinator (see Fig. A2.19)	Posterior interosseous nerve (radial nerve)	Posterior cord	Posterior division	Upper trunk		C5	C6		
Extensor carpi ulnaris (see Fig. A2.20)	Posterior interosseous nerve (radial nerve)	Posterior cord	Posterior division	Middle and lower trunk				C7	C8
Extensor digitorum (see Fig. A2.21)	Posterior interosseous nerve (radial nerve)	Posterior cord	Posterior division	Middle and lower trunk				C7	C8
Extensor digiti minimi (see Fig. A2.22)	Posterior interosseous nerve (radial nerve)	Posterior cord	Posterior division	Middle and lower				C7	C8
Abductor pollicis longus (see Fig. A2.23)	Posterior interosseous nerve (radial nerve)	Posterior cord	Posterior division	Middle and lower trunk				C7	C8
Extensor pollicis longus (see Fig. A2.24)	Posterior interosseous nerve (radial nerve)	Posterior cord	Posterior division	Middle and lower trunk				C7	C8
Extensor pollicis brevis (see Fig. A2.25)	Posterior interosseous nerve (radial nerve)	Posterior cord	Posterior division	Middle and lower trunk				C7	C8
Extensor indicis (see Fig. A2.26)	Posterior interosseous nerve (radial nerve)	Posterior cord	Posterior division	Middle and lower trunk				C7	C8

T1	Needle Insertion	Origin	Insertion	Action
	In a man, along the midaxillary line directly over the rib, anterior to the bulk of the latissimus dorsi; but, in a woman, posterior to breast tissue	At the outer surfaces and superior borders of the upper eighth or ninth rib	The medial border of the scapula, from the superior angle to the costal surface of the inferior angle	Protracts the scapula; assists upward rotation of the scapula
	At the mid arm level posterior to the lateral aspect of the shaft of the humerus	Long head, infraglenoid tubercle; lateral head, superior to the radial groove of the humerus; medial head, inferior to the radial groove	Posterior surface of the olecranon process of the ulna	Extends the forearm at the elbow
	2.5–3.75 cm distal to the olecranon along the radial border of the ulna	Lateral epicondyle of humerus	Olecranon and upper posterior surface of the ulna	Extends the forearm
	2–3 cm lateral to the biceps tendon	Lateral supracondylar ridge of the humerus	Base of the radial styloid process	Flexes the forearm at the elbow
	At the upper forearm 5–7.5 cm distal to the lateral epicondyle along a line connecting the epicondyle and the second metacarpal bone	The lower third of the lateral supracondylar ridge of the humerus	The radial surface of the base of the second and third metacarpal bone	Extends (dorsiflexion) and radially abducts the hand at the wrist
	With the forearm pronated, insert the needle 3–5 cm distal to the lateral epicondyle, toward the shaft of the radius	Lateral epicondyle, radial collateral, and annular ligaments	Lateral side of the upper part of the radius	Supinates the forearm
	The mid to upper forearm just radial to the lateral margin of the shaft of the ulna	The common extensor tendon from the lateral epicondyle of the humerus	At the ulnar side of the base of the fifth metacarpal bone	Extends (dorsiflexion) and ulnarly deviates the hand at wrist
	Dorsal side, mid forearm midway between the ulna and radius	Common extensor tendon from the lateral epicondyle of the humerus	The dorsal surface of all phalanges of second to fourth digits	Extends phalanges in second to fourth digits
	The mid forearm midway between the ulna and the radius	Common extensor tendon and the interosseous membrane	Extensor expansion, base of the middle and distal phalanges	Extends the little finger
	At the mid forearm along the shaft of the radius	Interosseous membrane, middle third of posterior surfaces of the radius and ulna	Lateral surface of the base of first metacarpal	Abducts the thumb radially
	At the mid forearm along the radial border of the ulna	Interosseous membrane and the middle third of the posterior surface of the ulna	Base of the distal phalanx of the thumb	Extends all parts of the thumb but specifically extends the distal phalanx; assists adduction of the thumb
	4–6 cm proximal to the wrist over the ulnar aspect of the radius	Interosseous membrane and posterior surface of the middle third of the radius	Base of the proximal phalanx of the thumb	Extends the proximal phalanx of the thumb
	5–7 cm proximal to the ulnar styloid just radial to the shaft of the ulna	Posterior surface of the ulna and interosseous membrane	Extensor expansion of the index finger	Extends the index finger

Continued

TABLE 5.4 ■ Common Muscles—Innervation, Location, and Needle Placement (See Video 5.1)—Cont'd

Muscle	Nerve	Cord	Division	Trunk	C4	C5	C6	C7	C8
Pronator teres (see Fig. A2.27 and Video 5.6)	Median nerve	Lateral cord	Anterior division	Upper and middle trunk			C6	C7	
Flexor carpi radialis (see Fig. A2.28)	Median nerve	Lateral cord	Anterior division	Upper and middle trunk			C6	C7	
Palmaris longus (see Fig. A2.29)	Median nerve	Lateral and medial cord	Anterior division	Middle and lower trunk				C7	C8
Flexor digitorum superficialis (see Fig. A2.30)	Median nerve	Lateral and medial cord	Anterior division	Middle and lower trunk				C7	C8
Flexor digitorum profundus (see Fig. A2.31)	Anterior interosseous nerve (median nerve) and ulnar nerve	Lateral and medial cord	Anterior division	Middle and lower trunk				C7	C8
Flexor pollicis longus (see Fig. A2.32)	Anterior interosseous nerve (median nerve)	Lateral and medial cord	Anterior division	Middle and lower trunk				C7	C8
Pronator quadratus (see Fig. A2.27)	Anterior interosseous nerve (median nerve)	Lateral and medial cord	Anterior division	Middle and lower trunk				C7	C8
Abductor pollicis brevis (see Fig. A2.33 and Video 5.7)	Median nerve	Medial cord	Anterior division	Lower trunk					C8
Flexor pollicis brevis (see Fig. A2.35)	Median nerve: superficial head. Ulnar nerve: deep head	Medial cord	Anterior division	Lower trunk					C8
Flexor carpi ulnaris (see Fig. A2.36)	Ulnar nerve	Medial cord	Anterior division	Lower trunk					C8

T1	Needle Insertion	Origin	Insertion	Action
	At 2–3 cm distal and 1 cm medial to the biceps tendon	Medial epicondyle and coronoid process of the ulna	Middle of the lateral side of the radius	Pronates the forearm
	The volar surface of the forearm 7–9 cm distal to the medial epicondyle along a line directed toward the muscle tendon at the wrist	Medial epicondyle of the humerus	Volar surface of the base of the second metacarpal	Flexes the hand at the wrist (palmar flexion); assists in radial abduction of the hand
T1	The volar surface of the forearm 6–8 cm distal to the medial epicondyle along a line directed toward the muscle tendon at the wrist	Medial epicondyle of the humerus	Flexor retinaculum, palmar aponeurosis	Flexes the hand at the wrist
T1	The volar surface of the forearm approximately 7–9 cm distal to the biceps tendon (mid forearm) and 2–3 cm medial to the ventral midline	Medial epicondyle of the humerus by the common tendon, coronoid process of ulna, and oblique line of the radius	The sides of the second phalanges of second to fifth digits	Flexes the proximal interphalangeal joints
T1	5–7.5 cm distal to the olecranon process and 1–1.5 cm medial to the shaft of the ulna	Anteromedial surface of ulna, interosseous membrane	Bases of the distal phalanges of the fingers	Flexes distal phalanges of the fingers; assists in flexion of the hand at the wrist
T1	5–7.5 cm proximal and 0–1.2 cm lateral to the radial artery pulse	Anterior surface of the radius, interosseous membrane, and coronoid process	Base of the distal phalanx of the thumb	Flexes the thumb, particularly the distal phalanx; assists in ulnar adduction of the thumb
T1	2.5 cm proximal to the ulnar styloid, midpoint between the radial and ulnar bones, deep to 2.5 cm to penetrate the interosseous membrane	The distal fourth of the volar surface of the ulna	The distal fourth of the lateral border and the volar surface of the radius	Pronates the forearm
T1	Obliquely near the muscle origin along the muscle	Flexor retinaculum, scaphoid, and trapezium	Lateral side of the base of the proximal phalanx of the thumb	Abducts the thumb
T1	Superficial head: a depth of 0.5–1 cm at the mid-point of a line drawn between the first meta-carpophalangeal joint and the pisiform. Deep head: the same as that for the superficial head, but insert the needle to a depth of 1–2 cm.	The superficial head originates in the flexor retinaculum and trapezium. The deep head originates in the ulnar aspect of the first metacarpal bone.	The superficial head is inserted at the radial aspect of the base of the proximal phalanx of the thumb. The deep head is inserted at the ulnar aspect of the base of the proximal phalanx of the thumb.	Flexes the proximal phalanx of thumb; assists in opposition, ulnar adduction (entire muscle), and palmar abduction (superficial head) of the thumb
T1	5–8 cm distal to the medial epicondyle along a line connecting the medial epicondyle and pisiform bone	Lateral epicondyle and posterior surface of ulna	Base of fifth metacarpal	Flexes and ulnarly deviates the hand at the wrist

Continued

TABLE 5.4 ■ **Common Muscles—Innervation, Location, and Needle Placement (See Video 5.1)—Cont'd**

Muscle	Nerve	Cord	Division	Trunk	C4	C5	C6	C7	C8
Abductor digiti minimi (see Fig. A2.37 and Video 5.8)	Ulnar nerve	Medial cord	Anterior division	Lower trunk					C8
Opponens digiti minimi (see Fig. A2.38)	Ulnar nerve	Medial cord	Anterior division	Lower trunk					C8
Flexor digiti minimi (see Fig. A2.39)	Ulnar nerve	Medial cord	Anterior division	Lower trunk					C8
Palmar interosseous (see Fig. A2.40)	Ulnar nerve	Medial cord	Anterior division	Lower trunk					C8
Dorsal interosseous (the first one) (see Fig. A2.41 and Video 5.9)	Ulnar nerve	Medial cord	Anterior division	Lower trunk					C8
Adduct or pollicis (see Fig. A2.42)	Ulnar nerve	Medial cord	Anterior division	Lower trunk					C8
Lumbricals (4) (see Fig. A2.43)	Median nerve (two lateral) and ulnar nerve (two medial)	Medial cord	Anterior division	Lower trunk					C8
Pectoralis major (see Fig. A2.44)	Lateral and medial pectoral nerves	Lateral cord	Anterior division	Upper, middle, and lower trunk		C5	C6	C7	C8
Pectoralis minor (see Fig. A2.44)	Medial pectoral nerve	Lateral cord	Anterior division	Upper, middle, and lower trunk		C5	C6	C7	C8

T1	Needle Insertion	Origin	Insertion	Action
T1	Insert the needle obliquely at the midpoint between the fifth metacarpophalangeal joint (metacarpophalangeal crease) and the ulnar aspect of the pisiform (distal wrist crease)	Pisiform and tendon of flexor carpi ulnaris	Pisiform and tendon of flexor carpi ulnaris	Abducts the little finger
T1	The midpoint between the fifth metacarpophalangeal joint (metacarpophalangeal crease) and the pisiform (distal wrist crease), just radial to the abductor digiti minimi	Flexor retinaculum and hook of hamate	Medial side of fifth metacarpal	Opposes the little finger
T1	The midpoint between the fifth metacarpophalangeal joint (metacarpophalangeal crease) and the ulnar aspect of the pisiform (distal wrist crease), just radial to the abductor digiti minimi	The hook of the hamate and the flexor retinaculum	The ulnar side of the base of the proximal phalanx of the little finger	Flexes the proximal phalanx of the fifth digit
T1	Just ulnar to the second metacarpal bone or just radial to the fourth and fifth metacarpal bones, respectively	Medial side of the second metacarpal; lateral sides of fourth and fifth metacarpals	Bases of the proximal phalanges in the same sides as their origins; extensor expansion	Adducts the fingers; flexes the metacarpophalangeal joints; extends interphalangeal joints
T1	Obliquely just proximal to the second metacarpophalangeal joint, and directed rostrally along the muscle belly	The ulnar border of the first metacarpal bone (outer head) and the radial border of the second metacarpal bone (inner head)	The radial aspect of the base of the proximal phalanx of the index finger	Abducts the index finger (radial deviation)
T1	The first web space just anterior (volar) to the edge of the first dorsal interosseous and proximal to the first metacarpophalangeal joint	Capitate and bases of second and third metacarpals (oblique head); palmar surface of the third metacarpal (transverse head)	Medial side of the base of the proximal phalanx of the thumb	Adducts the thumb
T1	Proximal to the metacarpophalangeal joint and radial to the flexor tendon	Lateral side of the tendons of the flexor digitorum profundus	Lateral side of the extensor expansion	Flexes the metacarpophalangeal joints and extends the interphalangeal joints
T1	Medial to the anterior axillary fold over the bulk of the muscle	The clavicular part originates at the sternal half of the clavicle. The sternocostal part originates at the anterior surface of the sternum, the edge of the first six or seven ribs, and the aponeurosis of the external oblique muscle of the abdomen.	The lateral lip of the intertubercular sulcus on the shaft of the humerus	Adducts and medially rotates the arm. Clavicular portion: assists in flexion of arm.
T1	The midclavicular line overlying the third rib	The outer surfaces of the third to fifth ribs (frequently second to fourth)	Coracoid process of the scapula	Depresses the shoulder

Continued

TABLE 5.4 ■ **Common Muscles—Innervation, Location, and Needle Placement (See Video 5.1)—Cont'd**

Muscle	Nerve	Division	L2	L3	L4	L5	S1	S2	S3
Iliopsoas (see Fig. A2.45)	Femoral nerve		L2	L3					
Sartorius (see Figs. A2.46 and A2.47)	Femoral nerve		L2	L3					
Rectus femoris (see Figs. A2.46 and A2.48)	Femoral nerve		L2	L3	L4				
Vastus lateralis (see Figs. A2.46 and A2.49)	Femoral nerve		L2	L3	L4				
Vastus intermedius (see Figs. A2.46 and A2.50)	Femoral nerve		L2	L3	L4				
Vastus medialis (see Figs. A2.46 and A2.51 and Video 5.10)	Femoral nerve		L2	L3	L4				
Pectineus (see Fig. A2.52)	Femoral nerve		L2	L3					
Adductor brevis (see Fig. A2.53)	Obturator nerve		L2	L3	L4				
Adductor longus (see Fig. A2.54)	Obturator nerve		L2	L3	L4				
Gracilis (see Fig. A2.55)	Obturator nerve		L2	L3	L4				
Adductor magnus (see Fig. A2.56)	Obturator and sciatic nerve		L2	L3	L4				
Gluteus medius (see Fig. A2.57)	Superior gluteal nerve	Posterior			L4	L5	S1		
Gluteus minimus (see Fig. A2.58)	Superior gluteal nerve	Posterior			L4	L5	S1		
Tensor fasciae latae (see Fig. A2.59)	Superior gluteal nerve	Posterior			L4	L5	S1		

Needle Insertion	Origin	Insertion	Action
3–4 cm lateral to the femoral artery pulse just below the inguinal ligament	Iliac fossa, ala of sacrum, and lumbar spine	Lesser trochanter on the shaft of the femur, anteromedially	Flexes and rotates the thigh medially
5–7.5 cm distal to the anterior superior iliac spine along a line to the medial epicondyle of the tibia	Anterior superior iliac spine	Upper medial side of tibia	Flexes and rotates thigh laterally; flexes and rotates leg medially
The anterior thigh midway between the anterior superior iliac spine and the patella	Anterior inferior iliac spine; posterior superior rim of acetabulum	Base of the patella; tibial tuberosity	Flexes the thigh; extends the leg
The anterolateral thigh 7.5–10 cm above the patella	Intertrochanteric line; greater trochanter; linea aspera; gluteal tuberosity; lateral intermuscular septum	Lateral side of the patella; tibial tuberosity	Extends the leg
The anterior thigh midway between the anterior superior iliac spine and the patella and under the rectus femoris	Upper shaft of the femur; lower lateral intermuscular septum	Upper border of the patella; tibial tuberosity	Extends the leg
The anteromedial thigh 5–7.5 cm above the patella	Intertrochanteric line; linea aspera; medial intermuscular septum	Medial side of the patella; tibial tuberosity	Extends the leg
2.5 cm medial to the femoral artery pulse just below the inguinal ligament	Superior ramus of the pubis	Along a line from the lesser trochanter to the linea aspera of the femur	Adducts and flexes the thigh
In the proximal one-sixth of the thigh, one-quarter the distance from the medial border to the anterior border of the thigh	Body and inferior pubic ramus	Pectineal line; upper part of linea aspera	Adducts, flexes, and rotates the thigh laterally
In the proximal one-fifth of the thigh, one-quarter the distance from the medial border to the anterior border of the thigh	Body of the pubis below its crest	Middle third of linea aspera	Adducts, flexes, and rotates the thigh laterally
The junction of the upper and middle thirds of the thigh, directly medial	Body and inferior pubic of the ramus	Medial surface of upper quarter of the tibia	Adducts and flexes the thigh; flexes and rotates the leg medially
Upper one-third of the thigh, immediately posterior to the medial border of the thigh	Ischiopubic ramus; ischial tuberosity	Linea aspera; medial supracondylar line; adductor tubercle	Adducts, flexes, and extends the thigh
2.5 centimeter distal to the midpoint of the iliac crest	Superolateral surface of the ilium	Greater trochanter	Abducts and aids medial rotation of thigh
Midway between the iliac crest and the greater trochanter of the femur	Ilium between the anterior and inferior gluteal lines	Greater trochanter	Abducts and aids medial rotation of the thigh
Midway between the anterior superior iliac spine and the greater trochanter of the femur	Iliac crest; anterior superior iliac spine	Iliotibial tract	Flexes, abducts, and rotates the thigh medially

Continued

TABLE 5.4 ■ Common Muscles—Innervation, Location, and Needle Placement (See Video 5.1)—Cont'd

Muscle	Nerve	Division	L2	L3	L4	L5	S1	S2	S3
Gluteus maximus (see Fig. A2.60)	Inferior gluteal nerve	Posterior				L5	S1	S2	
Semitendinosus (see Fig. A2.61)	Sciatic nerve	Tibial				L5	S1	S2	
Semimembranosus (see Fig. A2.62 and Video 5.11)	Sciatic nerve	Tibial				L5	S1	S2	
Biceps femoris (see Fig. A2.63 and Video 5.12)	Tibial nerve (long head) and common fibular nerve (short head) divisions of the sciatic nerve					L5	S1	S2	
Extensor digitorum longus (see Fig. A2.64)	Deep fibular nerve	Posterior				L5	S1		
Tibialis anterior (see Fig. A2.65 and Video 5.13)	Deep fibular nerve	Posterior			L4	L5			
Extensor hallucis longus (see Fig. A2.66)	Deep fibular nerve	Posterior				L5	S1		
Peroneus tertius (see Fig. A2.67)	Deep fibular nerve	Posterior				L5	S1		
Extensor digitorum brevis (see Fig. A2.68 and Video 5.14)	Deep fibular nerve	Posterior				L5	S1		
Peroneus longus (see Fig. A2.69)	Superficial fibular nerve	Fibular division of sciatic nerve				L5	S1		
Peroneus brevis (see Fig. A2.70)	Superficial fibular nerve	Fibular division of sciatic nerve				L5	S1		
Gastrocnemius (see Fig. A2.71 and Video 5.15)	Tibial nerve	Anterior					S1	S2	
Popliteus (see Fig. A2.72)	Tibial nerve	Anterior			L4	L5	S1		

Needle Insertion	Origin	Insertion	Action
Midpoint of the line connecting the posterior inferior iliac spine and greater trochanter	Posterosuperior ilium and sacrum	Gluteal tuberosity of the femur and iliotibial tract	Extends, abducts, and laterally rotates the thigh
One-third to midway along a line connecting the semitendinosus tendon (easily palpable as it forms the proximal medial margin of the popliteal fossa) with the ischial tuberosity	Ischial tuberosity	Medial surface of the upper part of the tibia	Extends the thigh; flexes and rotates the leg medially
Mid thigh, at or just medial to the midline and immediately subcutaneous	Ischial tuberosity	Medial condyle of the tibia	Extends the thigh; flexes and rotates the leg medially
Long head: one-third to midway along a line connecting the fibular head with the ischial tuberosity. Short head: palpate the tendon of the long head of the biceps femoris in the popliteal fossa. Insert the needle just medial to the tendon.	Long head from ischial tuberosity; short head from linea aspera and upper supracondylar line	Head of the fibula	Extends the thigh; flexes and rotates the leg medially
5–7.5 cm distal to the tibial tuberosity and 4–5 cm lateral to the shaft of the tibia	Lateral condyle of the tibia, interosseous membrane, and fibula	Bases of the middle and distal phalanges	Extends the toes; dorsiflexes the foot
Just lateral to the proximal half of the shaft of the tibia	Proximal half of the anterior tibial interosseous membrane and the lateral tibial condyle	Medial (first) cuneiform bone and the base of the first metatarsal	Dorsiflexes and inverts the ankle
7.5–8.75 cm proximal to the bimalleolar line of the ankle just lateral to the shaft of the tibia	Middle half of the anterior surface of the fibula; interosseous membrane	Base of the distal phalanx of the big toe	Extends the big toe; dorsiflexes and inverts the foot
6.5–7.5 cm proximal to the bimalleolar line of the ankle and 2–3 cm lateral to the shaft of the tibia	Distal one-third of fibula; interosseous membrane	Base of fifth metatarsal	Dorsiflexes and everts the foot
The superficial muscle tissue located on the proximal lateral aspect of the dorsum of the foot	Calcaneus	Extensor hood of second to fourth toes	Assists in the extension of all toes except the little toe
5–7.5 cm below the fibular head along the lateral aspect of the fibula	Lateral tibial condyle; head and upper lateral side of fibula	Medial cuneiform bone and base of first metatarsal	Everts and plantar flexes the foot
9–10 cm above the lateral malleolus just posterior to the lateral aspect of the fibula	Lower lateral side of the fibula; intermuscular septa	Base of the fifth metatarsal	Everts and plantar flexes the foot
The midpoint of the medial mass of the calf	Posterior surfaces of the lateral (lateral head) and medial (medial head) femoral condyles	Calcaneus	Plantar flexes the foot
The floor of the popliteal fossa in the proximal leg, midway between the insertions of the outer and inner hamstring tendons	Lateral femoral condyle	Medially on the proximal posterior tibia	Medially rotates and flexes the knee

Continued

TABLE 5.4 ■ Common Muscles—Innervation, Location, and Needle Placement (See Video 5.1)—Cont'd

Muscle	Nerve	Division	L2	L3	L4	L5	S1	S2	S3
Soleus (see Fig. A2.73)	Tibial nerve	Anterior					S1	S2	
Tibialis posterior (see Fig. A2.74)	Tibial nerve	Anterior			L4	L5	S1		
Flexor hallucis longus (see Fig. A2.75)	Tibial nerve	Anterior				L5	S1	S2	
Abductor digiti minimi (see Fig. A2.76)	Tibial nerve	Anterior					S1	S2	S3
Flexor digiti minimi (see Fig. A2.77)	Lateral plantar nerve of tibial nerve	Anterior					S1	S2	
Dorsal interossei (see Fig. A2.78)	Lateral plantar nerve (tibial nerve)							S2	S3
Plantar interossei (see Fig. A2.79)	Lateral plantar nerve (tibial nerve)	Anterior						S2	S3
Adductor hallucis (see Fig. A2.80)	Lateral plantar nerve (tibial nerve)	Anterior					S1	S2	S3
Abductor hallucis (see Fig. A2.81)	Medial plantar nerve (tibial nerve)	Anterior					S1	S2	
Flexor digitorum brevis (see Fig. A2.82)	Medial plantar nerve (tibial nerve)	Anterior					S1	S2	
Flexor hallucis brevis (see Fig. A2.83)	Medial plantar nerve (tibial nerve)	Anterior					S1	S2	

Paraspinal Muscles

Muscle	Spinal Nerve
Cervical paraspinal muscles (including multifidus, supraspinalis, interspinales, rectus capitis and obliquus capitis (see Fig. A2.84)	Posterior primary rami of cervical spinal nerves corresponding to the respective level. (Intermediate muscles may be innervated by multiple levels.)
Thoracic paraspinal muscles (see Fig. A2.85)	Posterior primary rami of thoracic spinal nerves corresponding to the respective level. (Intermediate muscles may be innervated by multiple levels.)
Lumbosacral paraspinal muscles (see Fig. A2.86)	Posterior primary rami of lumbar and sacral spinal nerves corresponding to the respective level. (Intermediate muscles may be innervated by multiple levels.)

Needle Insertion	Origin	Insertion	Action
Just distal to the belly of the medial gastrocnemius, medial to the Achilles tendon	Proximal tibia, interosseous membrane, and fibula	Calcaneus	Plantar flexes the ankle
1 cm medial to the margin of the tibia at the junction of the upper two-thirds with the lower third of the shaft. Direct the needle obliquely through the soleus and flexor digitorum muscles.	Posterior shafts of the tibia, fibula, and interosseous membrane	Navicular and medial cuneiform bones	Plantar flexes and inverts the foot
The posterolateral aspect of the lower leg, at the junction of the upper two-thirds and the lower third		Base of distal phalanx of the big toe	Flexes the distal phalanx of the big toe
Along the lateral border of the foot midway between the fifth metatarsal head and the calcaneus	Calcaneus	Lateral side of first phalanx of fifth toe	Abducts the fifth toe
On plantar aspect of the foot, midway between the cuboid and navicular bones	Base of the fifth metatarsal	Base of the first phalanx of the fifth toe	Flexes the proximal phalanx of the fifth toe
On dorsum of foot, between the metatarsals	Adjacent shafts of metatarsals	Proximal phalanges of second toes (medial and lateral sides), and third and fourth toes (lateral sides)	Abduct the toes; flex proximal, and extend the distal phalanges
On plantar aspect of the foot, between the metatarsals	Medial sides of the third to fifth metatarsals	Medial sides of the base of third to fifth proximal phalanges	Adduct the toes; flex proximal, and extend the distal phalanges
4–5 cm proximal to the second metatarsal head to a depth of 2 cm or more (the muscle lies deep); this will access the thick, fleshy oblique head	Oblique head: bases of the second to fourth metatarsals. Transverse head: capsule of the lateral four metatarsophalangeal joints.	Proximal phalanx of the big toe	Adducts the big toe
The muscle belly directly beneath the navicular bone	Medial tubercle of calcaneus	Base of the proximal phalanx of the big toe	Abducts the big toe
Midway between the third metatarsal head and the calcaneus	Medial tubercle of calcaneus	Middle phalanges of the lateral four toes	Flexes the middle phalanx of the second to fifth toes
The plantar surface of the foot 2.5 cm proximal to the first metatarsal head	Cuboid; third cuneiform	Proximal phalanx of the big toe	Flexes the big toe

Paraspinal Muscles

Needle Insertion	Action
2 cm lateral to the spinous process of the corresponding level. Note that the C7 level is the most prominent spinous process.	Extension of the head
2 cm lateral to the spinous process of the corresponding level	Extension of the back
2 cm lateral to the spinous process of the corresponding level. Note that the L3–L4 intervertebral level is approximately the level of the posterior, superior iliac crest.	Extension of the hip

TABLE 5.5 ■ Potentials Seen on Needle Testing

	Miniature Endplate Potentials (MEPPs)	Endplate Potentials (EPPs)	Fibrillation Potentials (Fibs)	Positive Sharp Waves (PSWs)	Fasciculation Potentials	Complex Repetitive Discharges (CRD)	Myotonic Discharges
Sound	Sea shells	Sputtering fat in a hot pan	Drops of rain on a tin roof	Dull thud	Varies	Misfired motor boat	Dive bomber
Firing pattern	Irregular	Irregular	Regular	Regular	Irregular	Regular/starts and stops abruptly	Waxes and wanes
Duration (msec)	1–2	3–5	1–5	10–30	5–15	Variable	>5–20
Amplitude (µV)	10–20	100–200	20–1000	20–1000	>500	50–500	20–300
Rate (Hz)	150	50–100	0.5–15	0.5–15	0.1–10	10–100	20–100
Waveform/ Deflection	Monophasic negative (upward)	Biphasic negative (upward)	Triphasic with initial positive (downward) deflection	Biphasic with initial positive (downward) deflection	Similar to motor unit action potential (MUAP)	Similar to MUAP, fibs, PSWs	Similar to EPPs, fibs, and PSWs
Cause	Miniature endplate potentials	Irregularly firing muscle fiber action potentials	Spontaneous depolarization of a muscle fiber	Spontaneous depolarization of a muscle fiber	Spontaneous involuntary discharge of single motor unit	Depolarization of single muscle fiber with ephaptic spread to adjacent denervated fibers	Spontaneous discharge of a muscle fiber
Indicates	Needle in the endplate	Needle in the endplate	Denervation (may be due to neurogenic, muscle disorder or disorders of the NMJ)	Denervation (may be due to neurogenic, muscle disorder or disorders of the NMJ)	Processes that affect the lower motor neuron. Also seen in benign fasciculations	Chronic neuropathic and myopathic disorders	Myotonic dystrophy, myotonia congenita and paramyotonia, some myopathies, hyperkalemic periodic paralysis, and rarely in denervation

CHAPTER 6

Injuries to Peripheral Nerves

Lyn D. Weiss

Injuries to peripheral nerves can be broken down into those affecting the myelin and those affecting the axons. It is important to remember, however, that rarely is the myelin involved without at least some involvement of the axon (and vice versa). Electrodiagnostic testing can determine what type of nerve injury exists, how severe the injury is, and where the injury is located.

The Seddon Classification of Nerve Injuries divides nerve injuries into three categories: neurapraxia, axonotmesis, and neurotmesis. *Neurapraxia* is defined as conduction block: only the myelin is affected. *Axonotmesis* refers to an injury affecting only the nerve's axons. The stroma (supporting connective tissue) is intact. *Neurotmesis* refers to a complete nerve injury involving the myelin, axon, and all supporting structures.

Demyelinating Injuries

Demyelinating injuries can slow electrical conduction over the entire length of the nerve (uniform demyelination), slow segments of the nerve (segmental demyelination), slow focal areas of the nerve (focal demyelination), or produce conduction block (when focal demyelination is so severe that nerve action potential cannot propagate across that segment). These changes are described below.

1. Uniform demyelination: the entire length of the nerve displays a slower conduction velocity. This is typically seen in hereditary disorders such as Charcot–Marie–Tooth disease.
2. Segmental demyelination: uneven degree of demyelination in different nerve fibers throughout the course of the nerve. This can produce variable slowing of different nerve fibers, which presents as temporal dispersion (Fig. 6.1). For example, in the same nerve some fibers may be conducting at 50 m/sec, some at 40 m/sec, and some at 30 m/sec. The sum will be a waveform that has lower amplitude but is more dispersed (wider). Remember that the sum of all the nerve fibers contributes to the shape of the compound muscle action potential (CMAP).
3. Focal nerve slowing: localized area of demyelination (with subsequent remyelination with immature myelin) causes nerve slowing, which presents as a decrease in conduction velocity across the lesion (Fig. 6.2). For example, if the myelin of the ulnar nerve at the elbow is constantly injured by repeated compression, the myelin will be compromised in that one area only. The nerve would conduct normally both above and below the elbow. Conduction velocity would be slowed across the area of demyelination. This slowing is due to the immature myelin conducting at a slower rate than normal myelin.
4. Conduction block: an area of focal demyelination that is so severe that the action potential cannot propagate through the area of demyelination. This presents as decreased amplitude with proximal stimulation because the affected nerve fibers cannot contribute to the amplitude. The distal CMAP amplitude is maintained because the nerve fiber distal to the block is intact (Fig. 6.3). For example, if there is a tourniquet applied to the upper arm and the focal demyelination is so severe that the action potential can no longer propagate,

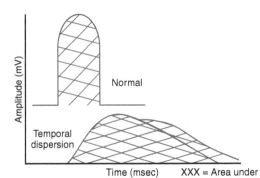

Fig. 6.1   Segmental demyelination.

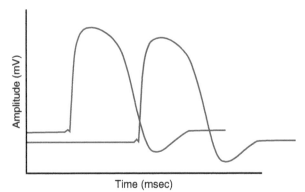

Fig. 6.2   Focal nerve slowing.

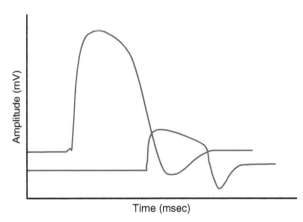

Fig. 6.3   Conduction block.

the CMAP obtained when stimulating proximal to this point will not include those affected nerve fibers and will therefore have a lower amplitude. However, when the nerve is stimulated distal to this area of compromise, the CMAP will be normal. This is because the axon itself has not been significantly compromised. Clinically, conduction blocks present as weakness. Conduction velocity slowing alone, without conduction block, does not produce clinical weakness.

The sum will be a waveform that has lower amplitude but is more dispersed (wider). As long as there is not a significant component of conduction block, the same number of axons are firing, and therefore the area under the curve remains the same. Remember that the sum of all of the nerve fibers contributes to the shape of the CMAP.

Axonal Injuries

Injury to the axon will lead to Wallerian degeneration distal to the site of the lesion. If the recording electrode is placed over a muscle distal to the lesion (i.e., one that has undergone Wallerian degeneration), you may see a decrease in CMAP amplitude with stimulation, both distal and proximal, to the lesion (Fig. 6.4; Fig. 6.5 shows a normal reading for comparison). On needle examination, abnormal spontaneous potentials (fibrillations [fibs] and positive sharp waves [PSWs]) may be noted acutely if the damage is severe enough. Depending on the chronicity of the injury, the motor unit action potentials (MUAPs) may be polyphasic with high amplitude and long duration. Recruitment of motor units may be decreased, and the firing frequency of single motor units will be increased. (Normal firing frequency for a MUAP is about 10 Hz or 10 cycles per second.)

Nerve Conduction Study and Electromyography Findings

See Table 6.1.

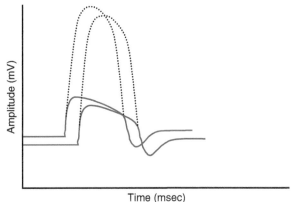

Fig. 6.4   Axonal neuropathy.

Time (msec)
(dotted line indicates normal amplitude)

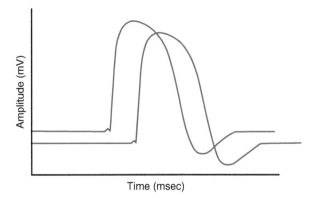

Fig. 6.5   Normal amplitude.

Time (msec)

TABLE 6.1 ■ NCS/EMG Findings in Peripheral Nerve Injuries

Condition	CMAP Amplitude With Distal Stimulation	CMAP Amplitude With Proximal Stimulation (Stimulating Across the Lesion)	Conduction Velocity	Distal Latency	Fibs/PSW	Recruitment
Uniform demyelinating	Normal	Normal	Decreased	Increased	−	Normal
Segmental demyelinating	Normal or decreased secondary to dispersion	Decreased secondary to dispersion	Decreased	May be increased (if fastest fibers are affected)	−	Normal
Focal demyelinating without conduction block[a]	Normal	Normal	Slowed across area of focal demyelination	Normal	−	Normal
Focal demyelination causing conduction block[a]	Normal	Decreased by more than 20%	Normal or focal slowing	Normal	−	Decreased
Axonotmesis	Decreased	Decreased	Normal to 20% decrease	Normal to 20% increase	+	Decreased
Neurotmesis	Unobtainable	Unobtainable	Unobtainable	Unobtainable	++	Unobtainable

[a]For the purposes of this table, assume a proximal area of focal demyelination or conduction block.
CMAP, Compound muscle action potential; EMG, electromyographic; fib, fibrillation potential; NCS, nerve conduction study; PSW, positive sharp wave.

NERVE CONDUCTION STUDIES

Demyelinating Injuries

Uniform Demyelinating. In uniform demyelinating lesions, nerve conduction studies (NCSs) will be slowed throughout the nerve because the entire nerve is affected. Distal latencies will be prolonged, again because of the uniform slowing (distal latencies representing the most distal conduction velocity). Amplitudes should not be significantly affected, because the axons are intact and the slowing is consistent through all fibers of the nerve.

Segmental Demyelination. Because there is variable slowing of different nerve fibers within the nerve, conduction velocity will be slowed and distal latencies will be prolonged in segmentally demyelinating injuries. CMAP amplitudes may be decreased because of temporal dispersion, not because of axonal damage. Therefore, the CMAP may be longer in duration. However, the area under the CMAP will be normal.

Focal Demyelination. In focal demyelination, only one segment of the nerve is affected. Therefore, conduction velocity will be normal unless stimulation is across the area of focal demyelination. In this segment, you will see slowing of conduction velocity. Slowing is usually evident if there is a more than 10 m/sec drop in conduction velocity across the segment, compared to the distal or proximal segments. Distal latencies and all amplitudes should be normal.

Conduction Block. As stated earlier, conduction block is a focal demyelination that is so severe that the action potential cannot propagate past that point. Therefore, distal latencies and conduction velocities remain normal. Distal amplitudes will be normal. However, when the nerve is stimulated across the area of conduction block, a drop in amplitude is noted. To be considered significant, this drop in proximal amplitude should be more than 20% of the distal amplitude. For example, if the distal amplitude is 10 µV and the proximal amplitude is 7 µV, conduction block should be considered.

Axonal Injuries

NCSs in axonal injuries will show decreased amplitude with both proximal and distal stimulation. If the contralateral extremity is not affected, you can compare side-to-side amplitudes to estimate the amount of axonal loss. Usually, a 50% side-to-side difference is considered significant. Latencies and conduction velocities should not be significantly affected. Sometimes, because the fastest fibers may be affected, a less than 20% increase in latency or decrease in conduction velocity may be noted. If neurotmesis is present, the CMAP or sensory nerve action potential (SNAP) amplitude will be unobtainable both proximal and distal to the lesion.

Electromyography Findings

Abnormal spontaneous potentials (fibrillations and PSWs) are usually only found when there has been axonal injury. Therefore, no abnormal spontaneous activity should be noted in any of the demyelinating lesions. MUAP morphology and recruitment should be normal. The only exception would be in conduction block, where decreased recruitment would be seen.

With Wallerian degeneration, the degeneration occurs distal to the site of the lesion. Therefore, all distal muscles innervated by the injured nerve should show spontaneous activity if the test is performed before reinnervation occurs. Polyphasicity, prolonged duration, and increased amplitude of the MUAP may be noted with chronic lesions, again depending upon the timing of the test. Recruitment will be decreased. In a neurotmetic lesion, there will be profound denervation and no motor units will be recruited.

Timing of Electrodiagnostic Testing: When to Schedule an EMG/NCS

To get the most information with the least amount of discomfort to the patient, it is important to time the test appropriately. Keep in mind the following timetable regarding how nerves respond electrophysiologically to injury:

1. Abnormal spontaneous activity includes fibrillation potentials (fibs) and PSWs. Such findings may take days to weeks before being detectable on needle electromyographic (EMG) testing. The more distal the muscle, the longer the axon length, and the longer it takes for membrane instability to occur. Proximal muscles may show changes within 1 week, but collateral sprouting will also provide reinnervation to these muscles first. More distal muscles may require 3 weeks before fibs or PSWs are seen. Therefore, if the test is done too early (e.g., in the first few weeks after injury), it may be falsely negative. If a test is performed long after the injury, reinnervation may have already occurred. In this case, there may not be fibs and PSWs present. Motor units may show evidence of reinnervation: long duration, polyphasic, and increased amplitude. For purposes of timing the study, the time of the injury should be considered the time of the initial presentation of signs or symptoms of nerve involvement, as scarring or late effects of a traumatic injury may not correspond to the initial time of an injury.

2. SNAP and CMAP amplitudes begin to decrease within several days after nerve injury. It may take over 1 week before SNAPs and CMAPs are unobtainable. Therefore, if NCS are done in the first few days after injury, they may appear normal when, in fact, if they were done at least 11 days following the injury, they would reveal reduced amplitudes consistent with the suspected injury.

3. Axons regrow at a rate of about 1 mm/day (about 1 inch/month). Therefore, if you are doing a study or serial studies where you want to determine the prognosis, it is important to keep in mind how long the anticipated recovery period would be based on axonal regeneration.

CHAPTER 7

How to Plan Out the Examination

Lyn D. Weiss

To perform electrodiagnostic testing accurately and efficiently, a well-planned approach is necessary. Such measures will decrease potential discomfort and increase the yield of information. The clinician should start by taking a thorough history, performing a physical examination, and, if available, reviewing laboratory and radiologic studies. Electrodiagnostic testing serves as an extension of the history and physical examination in the evaluation of neuromuscular disease and pathology. Although the nature of neurologic dysfunction in a specific disease process may be suggested by symptoms or signs obtained during physical examination, only electrodiagnostic studies can provide objective physiologic measures of neurologic functions.

Once the history and physical are performed, you should develop a differential diagnosis that will help guide which nerves and muscles you decide to test. There are several questions that can help you narrow your selections (Fig. 7.1).

- Are the symptoms compatible with a central disorder (hyperreflexia, increased tone, central distribution) or a peripheral disorder (hyporeflexia, decreased tone, peripheral distribution)? If the history and physical are compatible with a central disorder, other testing may be more appropriate (i.e., magnetic resonance imaging [MRI] of the brain or spinal cord). If a peripheral distribution is suggested, proceed with electromyography (EMG) and/or nerve conduction studies (NCSs).
- Does the history and physical suggest a disorder of nerves (neuropathic) or muscles (myopathic)? A neuropathic disorder may present with sensory findings and/or weakness in a peripheral nerve distribution. A myopathic disorder should be considered if there is predominantly proximal weakness and no sensory symptoms (see Chapter 17, Myopathy).
- If a neuropathic disorder is more likely, try to determine if the motor and sensory loss reflects a peripheral neuropathy (predominantly distal affecting more than one extremity) or a mononeuropathy.
- If a peripheral nerve lesion is probable, use Table 7.1 to try to localize the lesion. Table 7.1 will help you identify the patient's symptoms, depending on whether the problem is at the root, trunk, cord division, or peripheral nerve level. It will also help you determine which nerves and muscles should be tested.
- If a peripheral neuropathy is suspected, electrodiagnostic testing will help determine the type of neuropathy (motor and/or sensory; axonal and/or demyelinating).

General Points

- If you get an abnormal result, it is important to continue testing until you get a normal result. For example, if you suspect carpal tunnel syndrome and needle testing of the abductor pollicis brevis (APB) is abnormal (fibrillations or positive sharp waves are present), other

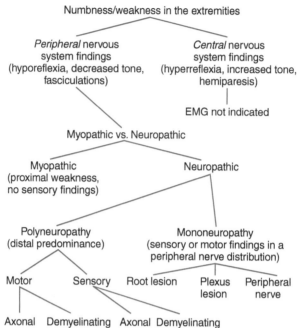

Fig. 7.1 Algorithm for planning the electrodiagnostic examination.

muscles should be tested. A more proximal median neuropathy or a generalized disorder may be present.
- To assess for peripheral neuropathy, motor and sensory nerves in three extremities should be tested.
- When performing needle testing to rule out local nerve injury or entrapment, start with the most distally innervated muscles and proceed proximally.
- If the patient is reluctant to proceed with the electrodiagnostic test, go directly to that portion of the test that is most likely to yield pertinent information. For example, some electromyographers have a prescribed list and schedule of nerves to test. While this may suffice for 90% of patients, flexibility is necessary if you know the patient can tolerate only limited testing.

Table 7.1 shows commonly tested nerves in the upper and lower extremities, the root levels, the muscles they innervate, and some of the physical findings that can be expected if the nerve is compromised. This table can be used to help plan out the electrodiagnostic test. Table 7.2 describes common muscles tested on needle study, along with nerve and root levels. This will assist with planning out the examination. For example, if a C6 nerve root lesion is suspected, try to examine several muscles that include C6. If a radial nerve injury is suspected, these tables will help decide which muscles to test based on their innervation.

TABLE 7.1 ■ Upper Extremities

Roots	Nerves	Muscles	Root Lesion Signs and Symptoms
C5	Dorsal scapular	Rhomboid major	Weakness or absent scapula adduction
	Dorsal scapular	Rhomboid minor	Weakness in shoulder range of motion
	Dorsal scapular	Levator scapulae	Weakness in arm abduction, adduction, flexion, and medial/lateral rotation
	Suprascapular	Supraspinatus	Weakness in flexion of forearm at elbow and supination of forearm
	Suprascapular	Infraspinatus	Diminished sensation over the lateral arm
	Subscapular	Subscapularis	
	Subscapular	Teres major	
	Axillary	Deltoid	
	Axillary	Teres minor	
	Musculocutaneous	Coracobrachialis	
	Musculocutaneous	Biceps	
	Musculocutaneous	Brachialis	
	Long thoracic	Serratus anterior	
	Radial	Brachioradialis	
	Radial	Supinator	
	Pectoral	Pectoralis major	
	Pectoral	Pectoralis minor	

Continued

—cont'd

TABLE 7.1 ■ Upper Extremities

Roots	Nerves	Muscles	Root Lesion Signs and Symptoms
C6	Suprascapular	Supraspinatus	Weakness in arm abduction, adduction, flexion and medial/lateral rotation
	Suprascapular	Infraspinatus	Weakness in extension/flexion of forearm at elbow and pronation of forearm
	Subscapular	Subscapularis	Weakness in extension (dorsiflexion) of wrist and radial abduction of hand at wrist
	Subscapular	Teres major	Diminished sensation over the lateral forearm, thumb, index, and one-half of middle finger (radial side)
	Axillary	Deltoid	
	Axillary	Teres minor	
	Musculocutaneous	Biceps	
	Musculocutaneous	Brachialis	
	Musculocutaneous	Coracobrachialis	
	Thoracodorsal	Latissimus dorsi	
	Long thoracic	Serratus anterior	
	Radial	Triceps	
	Radial	Anconeus	
	Radial	Brachioradialis	
	Radial	Extensor carpi radialis	
	Radial	Supinator	
	Median	Pronator teres	
	Median	Flexor carpi radialis	
	Pectoral	Pectoralis major	
	Pectoral	Pectoralis minor	

	Nerve	Muscle	Clinical finding
C7	Subscapular	Teres major	
	Musculocutaneous	Coracobrachialis	Weak or absent extension of forearm at elbow and pronation of forearm
			Unable to flex (palmar flexion) hand at wrist and extend fingers at metacarpophalangeal (MCP) joint
	Thoracodorsal	Latissimus dorsi	Inability to dorsiflex the wrist and ulnar deviation
	Long thoracic	Serratus anterior	Weakness in extension (dorsiflexion) of wrist and radial abduction of hand at wrist
	Radial	Triceps	Weakness in extension of proximal and distal phalanx of thumb
	Radial	Anconeus	Diminished sensation over middle finger
	Radial	Extensor carpi radialis	
	Radial	Extensor carpi ulnaris	
	Radial	Extensor digitorum	
	Radial	Extensor digiti minimi	
	Radial	Abductor pollicis longus	
	Radial	Extensor pollicis longus	
	Radial	Extensor pollicis brevis	
	Radial	Extensor indicis	
	Median	Pronator teres	
	Median	Flexor carpi radialis	
	Median	Palmaris longus	
	Median	Flexor digitorum superficialis	
	Median and ulnar	Flexor digitorum profundus	
	Median	Flexor pollicis longus	
	Median	Pronator quadratus	
	Pectoral	Pectoralis major	
	Pectoral	Pectoralis minor	

Continued

TABLE 7.1 ■ Upper Extremities—cont'd

Roots	Nerves	Muscles	Root Lesion Signs and Symptoms
C8	Radial	Extensor carpi ulnaris	Weakness in flexion of distal phalanges of fingers
	Radial	Extensor digitorum	Inability to adduct index, ring, and little fingers toward middle finger
	Radial	Extensor digiti minimi	Difficulty of abduction of index, middle, and ring fingers from middle line of middle finger, both radial and ulnar abduction
	Radial	Abductor pollicis longus	
	Radial	Extensor pollicis longus	Weakness in flexion and ulnar deviation of hand at wrist
	Radial	Extensor pollicis brevis	Weakness in abduction, flexion, and opposition of little finger toward thumb
	Radial	Extensor indicis	Unable to adduct the thumb in both ulnar and palmar directions
	Median	Palmaris longus	Diminished sensation over the distal half of the forearm's ulnar side, and the fifth and half of the
	Median	Flexor digitorum superficialis	fourth finger on the ulnar side
	Median and ulnar	Flexor digitorum profundus	
	Median	Flexor pollicis longus	
	Median	Pronator quadratus	
	Median	Abductor pollicis brevis	
	Median	Opponens pollicis	
	Median	Flexor pollicis brevis	
	Ulnar	Flexor carpi ulnaris	
	Ulnar	Palmaris brevis	
	Ulnar	Abductor digiti minimi	
	Ulnar	Opponens digiti minimi	
	Ulnar	Flexor digiti minimi	
	Ulnar	Palmar interosseous	
	Ulnar	Dorsal interosseous	
	Ulnar	Adductor pollicis	
	Median and ulnar	Lumbricals (4)	
	Pectoral	Pectoralis major	
	Pectoral	Pectoralis minor	

	Nerve	Muscle	Finding
T1	Median	Palmaris longus	Weakness in finger abduction Difficulty of abduction of index, middle, and ring fingers from middle line of middle finger; both radial and ulnar abduction
	Median	Flexor digitorum superficialis	
	Median and ulnar	Flexor digitorum profundus	Inability to adduct index, ring, and little fingers toward middle finger
	Median	Flexor pollicis longus	Weakness in little finger abduction, flexion and opposition of little finger toward thumb
	Median	Pronator quadratus	Weakness in adduction of the thumb in both ulnar and palmar directions and abduction of thumb
	Median	Abductor pollicis brevis	
	Median	Opponens pollicis	Diminished sensation over the medial side of the upper half of the forearm and the lower half of the arm
	Median	Flexor pollicis brevis	
	Ulnar	Flexor carpi ulnaris	
	Ulnar	Palmaris brevis	
	Ulnar	Abductor digiti minimi	
	Ulnar	Opponens digiti minimi	
	Ulnar	Flexor digiti minimi	
	Ulnar	Palmar interosseous	
	Ulnar	Dorsal interosseous	
	Ulnar	Adductor pollicis	
	Median and ulnar	Lumbricals (4)	
	Pectoral	Pectoralis major	
	Pectoral	Pectoralis minor	

Continued

TABLE 7.1 ■ Upper Extremities—cont'd

Trunks	Nerves	Muscles	Trunk Lesion Signs and Symptoms
Upper trunk C5, C6	Dorsal scapula	Rhomboid major	Weakness of shoulder and upper arm abduction, flexion, and external rotation
	Dorsal scapula	Rhomboid minor	Weakness in elbow flexion and radial wrist extension
	Dorsal scapula	Levator scapulae	Sensory loss at the C5 and C6 dermatomes—the lateral arm, forearm, and first two digits
	Suprascapular	Supraspinatus	
	Suprascapular	Infraspinatus	
	Suprascapular	Subscapularis	
	Suprascapular	Teres major	
	Axillary	Deltoid	
	Axillary	Teres minor	
	Musculocutaneous	Coracobrachialis	
	Musculocutaneous	Biceps	
	Musculocutaneous	Brachialis	
	Thoracodorsal	Latissimus dorsi	
	Radial	Triceps	
	Radial	Anconeus	
	Radial	Brachioradialis	
	Radial	Extensor carpi radialis	
	Radial	Supinator	
	Median	Pronator teres	
	Median	Flexor carpi radialis	
	Pectoral	Pectoralis major	
	Pectoral	Pectoralis minor	

	Nerve	Muscle	Clinical finding
Middle trunk C7	Musculocutaneous	Coracobrachialis	
	Thoracodorsal	Latissimus dorsi	
	Radial	Triceps	Weak or absent extension of forearm at elbow
	Radial	Anconeus	
	Radial	Extensor carpi radialis	Weak/absent extension (dorsiflexion) and radial abduction of hand at wrist Unable to flex (palmar flexion) hand at wrist and extend fingers at MCP
	Radial	Extensor carpi ulnaris	Inability to dorsiflex the wrist and ulnar deviation
	Radial	Extensor digitorum	Weak or absent extension of proximal and distal phalanx of thumb
	Radial	Extensor digiti minimi	Diminished sensation over middle finger and sometimes the index finger
	Radial	Abductor pollicis longus	
	Radial	Extensor pollicis longus	
	Radial	Extensor pollicis brevis	
	Radial	Extensor indicis	
	Median	Pronator teres	
	Median	Flexor carpi radialis	
	Median	Palmaris longus	
	Median	Flexor digitorum superficialis	
	Median and ulnar	Flexor digitorum profundus	
	Median	Flexor pollicis longus	
	Median	Pronator quadratus	
	Pectoral	Pectoralis major	
	Pectoral	Pectoralis minor	

Continued

TABLE 7.1 ■ Upper Extremities—cont'd

Trunks	Nerves	Muscles	Trunk Lesion Signs and Symptoms
Lower trunk C8, T1	Thoracodorsal	Latissimus dorsi	Weak or absent abduction, flexion, and opposition of little finger toward thumb
	Radial	Triceps	Inability to adduct index, ring, and little fingers toward middle finger
	Radial	Anconeus	Difficulty of abduction of index, middle, and ring fingers from middle line of middle finger, both radial and ulnar abduction
	Radial	Extensor carpi ulnaris	Unable to adduct the thumb in both ulnar and palmar directions
	Radial	Extensor digitorum	Weakness in extension of forearm and flexion of distal phalanges
	Radial	Extensor digiti minimi	Diminished sensation over distal half of the forearm ulnar side and the fifth and half of the fourth fingers on the ulnar side
	Radial	Abductor pollicis longus	
	Radial	Extensor pollicis longus	
	Radial	Extensor pollicis brevis	
	Radial	Extensor indicis	
	Median	Palmaris longus	
	Median	Flexor digitorum superficialis	
	Median and ulnar	Flexor digitorum profundus	
	Median	Flexor pollicis longus	
	Median	Pronator quadratus	
	Ulnar	Abductor digiti minimi	
	Ulnar	Opponens digiti minimi	
	Ulnar	Flexor digiti minimi	
	Ulnar	Palmar interosseous	
	Ulnar	Dorsal interosseous	
	Ulnar	Adductor pollicis	
	Median and ulnar	Lumbricals (4)	
	Pectoral	Pectoralis major	
	Pectoral	Pectoralis minor	

Cords	Nerves	Muscles	Cord Lesion Signs and Symptoms
Posterior cord C5–T1	Subscapular	Subscapularis	Weakness in shoulder range of motion (ROM) and arm abduction, adduction, flexion, extension, and lateral rotation
	Subscapular	Teres major	
	Axillary	Deltoid	Weak or absent extension of forearm at elbow
	Axillary	Teres minor	Weak or absent extension (dorsiflexion) and radial abduction of hand at wrist
	Thoracodorsal	Latissimus dorsal	Unable to supinate and extend fingers at MCP
	Radial	Triceps	Inability to dorsiflex the wrist and ulnar deviation
	Radial	Anconeus	Weak or absent extension of proximal and distal phalanx of thumb
	Radial	Brachioradialis	Diminished sensation over the lateral arm—deltoid patch on upper arm, lateral forearm, and first three digits
	Radial	Extensor carpi radialis	
	Radial	Supinator	
	Radial	Extensor carpi ulnaris	
	Radial	Extensor digitorum	
	Radial	Extensor digiti minimi	
	Radial	Abductor pollicis longus	
	Radial	Extensor pollicis longus	
	Radial	Extensor pollicis brevis	
	Radial	Extensor indicis	
Lateral cord C5–T1	Musculocutaneous	Coracobrachialis	Unable to pronate and flex the forearm
	Musculocutaneous	Biceps	Weakness in flexion of forearms and the hand at wrist
	Musculocutaneous	Brachialis	Weakness in flexion of distal phalanges of fingers
	Median	Pronator teres	Diminished sensation over the lateral forearm and middle finger
	Median	Flexor carpi radialis	
	Median	Palmaris longus	
	Median	Flexor digitorum superficialis	
	Median and ulnar	Flexor digitorum profundus	
	Median	Flexor pollicis longus	
	Pectoral	Pectoralis major	
	Pectoral	Pectoralis minor	

Continued

TABLE 7.1 ■ Upper Extremities—cont'd

Cords	Nerves	Muscles	Cord Lesion Signs and Symptoms
Medial cord C6–T1	Median	Palmaris longus	Weakness in flexion of distal phalanges of fingers
	Median	Flexor digitorum superficialis	Weak/absent abduction, flexion, and opposition of little finger toward thumb
	Median and ulnar	Flexor digitorum profundus	Inability to adduct index, ring, and little fingers toward middle finger
	Median	Flexor pollicis longus	Difficulty of abduction of index, middle, and ring fingers from middle line of middle finger, both radial and ulnar abduction
	Median	Pronator quadratus	
	Median	Abductor pollicis brevis	Unable to adduct the thumb in both ulnar and palmar directions
	Median	Opponens pollicis	Decreased sensation over the volar surface of the first, second, third, and half of the fourth fingers
	Median	Flexor pollicis brevis	
	Ulnar	Flexor carpi ulnaris	
	Ulnar	Palmaris brevis	
	Ulnar	Abductor digiti minimi	
	Ulnar	Opponens digiti minimi	
	Ulnar	Flexor digiti minimi	
	Ulnar	Palmar interosseous	
	Ulnar	Dorsal interosseous	
	Ulnar	Adductor pollicis	
	Median and ulnar	Lumbricals (4)	

Divisions	Nerves	Muscles	Division Lesion Signs and Symptoms
Posterior division C5–C8	Subscapular	Subscapularis	Weakness in shoulder ROM and arm abduction, adduction, flexion, extension, and lateral rotation
	Subscapular	Teres major	Weak or absent extension of forearm at elbow
	Axillary	Deltoid	Weak or absent extension (dorsiflexion) and radial abduction of hand at wrist
	Axillary	Teres minor	Unable to supinate and extend fingers at MCP
	Thoracodorsal	Latissimus dorsi	Inability to dorsiflex the wrist and ulnar deviation
	Radial	Triceps	Weak or absent extension of proximal and distal phalanx of thumb
	Radial	Anconeus	Diminished sensation over the lateral arm — deltoid patch on upper arm, lateral forearm, and first three digits
	Radial	Brachioradialis	
	Radial	Extensor carpi radialis	
	Radial	Supinator	
	Radial	Extensor carpi ulnaris	
	Radial	Extensor digitorum	
	Radial	Extensor digiti minimi	
	Radial	Abductor pollicis longus	
	Radial	Extensor pollicis longus	
	Radial	Extensor pollicis brevis	
	Radial	Extensor indicis	

Continued

TABLE 7.1 ■ Upper Extremities—cont'd

Divisions	Nerves	Muscles	Division Lesion Signs and Symptoms
Anterior division C5–T1	Musculocutaneous	Coracobrachialis	Weakness or absent supination of forearm and flexion of forearm at elbow
	Musculocutaneous	Biceps	Numbness/tingling sensation on the volar surface of the first, second, third, and half of the fourth fingers
	Musculocutaneous	Brachialis	
	Median	Pronator teres	Weak/absent palmar abduction of thumb (perpendicular to plane of palm)
	Median	Flexor carpi radialis	Weakness in flexion of distal phalanges of fingers
	Median	Palmaris longus	Weak/absent abduction, flexion, and opposition of little finger toward thumb
	Median	Flexor digitorum superficialis	Inability to adduct index, ring, and little fingers toward middle finger
	Median and ulnar	Flexor digitorum profundus	Difficulty of abduction of index, middle, and ring fingers from middle line of middle finger, both radial and ulnar abduction
	Median	Flexor pollicis longus	
	Median	Pronator quadratus	Unable to adduct the thumb in both ulnar and palmar directions
	Median	Abductor pollicis brevis	Diminished sensation over the lateral forearm and the third, fourth, and fifth fingers
	Median	Opponens pollicis	
	Median	Flexor pollicis brevis	
	Ulnar	Flexor carpi ulnaris	
	Ulnar	Palmaris brevis	
	Ulnar	Abductor digiti minimi	
	Ulnar	Opponens digiti minimi	
	Ulnar	Flexor digiti minimi	
	Ulnar	Palmar interosseous	
	Ulnar	Dorsal interosseous	
	Ulnar	Adductor pollicis	
	Median and ulnar	Lumbricals (4)	
	Pectoral	Pectoralis major	
	Pectoral	Pectoralis minor	

Peripheral Nerves	Roots	Muscles	Peripheral Nerve Lesion Signs and Symptoms
Axillary	C5, C6 C5, C6	Deltoid Teres minor	Weakness in shoulder range of motion and arm abduction, adduction, flexion, extension, and lateral rotation Diminished sensation over the lateral arm—deltoid patch on upper arm
Musculocutaneous	C5, C6, C7 C5, C6 C5, C6	Coracobrachialis Biceps Brachialis	Weakness or absent supination of forearm and flexion of forearm at elbow Decreased sensory over the lateral forearm
Radial	C6, C7, C8 C6, C7, C8 C5, C6 C6, C7 C5, C6 C7, C8 C7, C8 C7, C8 C7, C8 C7, C8 C7, C8 C7, C8	Triceps Anconeus Brachioradialis Extensor carpi radialis Supinator Extensor carpi ulnaris Extensor digitorum Extensor digiti minimi Abductor pollicis longus Extensor pollicis longus Extensor pollicis brevis Extensor indicis	Weak or absent extension of forearm at elbow Weak or absent extension (dorsiflexion) and radial abduction of hand at wrist Unable to supinate and extend fingers at MCP Inability to dorsiflex the wrist and ulnar deviation Weak or absent extension of proximal and distal phalanx of thumb Sensation is diminished over the web space between thumb and index finger

Continued

TABLE 7.1 ■ Upper Extremities—cont'd

Peripheral Nerves	Roots	Muscles	Peripheral Nerve Lesion Signs and Symptoms
Median	C6, C7	Pronator teres	Unable to pronate the forearm and flex the hand at wrist
	C6, C7	Flexor carpi radialis	Numbness/tingling sensation on the volar surface of the first, second, third, and half of the fourth fingers
	C7, C8, T1	Palmaris longus	Weak/absent palmar abduction of thumb (perpendicular to plane of palm)
	C7, C8, T1	Flexor digitorum superficialis	Unable to do the "OK" sign
	C7, C8, T1	Flexor digitorum profundus	Decreased sensation over the distal radial aspect index finger
	C7, C8, T1	Flexor pollicis longus	
	C7, C8, T1	Pronator quadratus	
	C8, T1	Abductor pollicis brevis	
	C8, T1	Opponens pollicis	
	C8, T1	Flexor pollicis brevis	
	C8, T1	Lumbricals	
Ulnar nerve	C8, T1	Flexor carpi ulnaris	Weak/absent abduction, flexion, and opposition of little finger toward thumb
	C8, T1	Flexor digitorum profundus	Inability to adduct index, ring, and little fingers toward middle finger
	C8, T1	Palmaris brevis	Difficulty of abduction of index, middle, and ring fingers from middle line of middle finger, both radial and ulnar abduction
	C8, T1	Abductor digiti minimi	Unable to adduct the thumb in both ulnar and palmar directions
	C8, T1	Opponens digiti minimi	Decreased sensory over the fifth and half of the fourth fingers on the ulnar side
	C8, T1	Flexor digiti minimi	
	C8, T1	Palmar interosseous	
	C8, T1	Dorsal interosseous	
	C8, T1	Adductor pollicis	
	C8, T1	Flexor pollicis brevis	
	C8, T1	Lumbricals	

Lower Extremities Root Lesion Signs and Symptoms

Roots	Nerves	Muscles	Lower Extremities Root Lesion Signs and Symptoms
L2	Femoral	Iliopsoas	Weakness in hip adduction and flexion
	Femoral	Sartorius	Weak or absent thigh adduction, flexion, and medial and lateral rotation
	Femoral	Rectus femoris	Weakness or inability to extend the leg at the knee
	Femoral	Vastus lateralis	Diminished sensation over the anterior and medial aspects of the thigh and in the
	Femoral	Vastus intermedius	medial aspect of the leg
	Femoral	Vastus medialis	
	Femoral	Pectineus	
	Obturator	Adductor brevis	
	Obturator	Adductor longus	
	Obturator	Gracilis	
	Obturator	Adductor magnus	
L3	Femoral	Iliopsoas	Weakness in hip adduction and flexion
	Femoral	Sartorius	Weak or absent thigh adduction, flexion, medial and lateral rotation
	Femoral	Rectus femoris	Weakness or inability to extend the leg at the knee
	Femoral	Vastus lateralis	Diminished sensation over the anterior and medial aspect of the thigh and knee
	Femoral	Vastus intermedius	
	Femoral	Vastus medialis	
	Femoral	Pectineus	
	Obturator	Adductor brevis	
	Obturator	Adductor longus	
	Obturator	Gracilis	
	Obturator	Adductor magnus	

Continued

TABLE 7.1 ■ Upper Extremities—cont'd

Roots	Nerves	Muscles	Lower Extremities Root Lesion Signs and Symptoms
L4	Femoral	Rectus femoris	Weakness in hip adduction and abduction
	Femoral	Vastus lateralis	Weak or absent thigh adduction, abduction, flexion, medial and lateral rotation
	Femoral	Vastus intermedius	Weakness in knee flexion, medial rotation, and extension
	Femoral	Vastus medialis	Loss of dorsiflexion (drop foot)
	Obturator	Adductor brevis	Limited inversion of foot
	Obturator	Adductor longus	Diminished sensation over the medial side of the distal leg and medial malleolus area
	Obturator	Gracilis	
	Obturator	Adductor magnus	
	Superior gluteal	Gluteus medius	
	Superior gluteal	Gluteus minimus	
	Superior gluteal	Tensor fasciae latae	
	Deep fibular	Tibialis anterior	
	Tibial	Popliteus	
L5	Superior gluteal	Gluteus medius	Weakness in adduction, abduction, flexion, extension, and medial and lateral rotation of thigh
	Superior gluteal	Gluteus minimus	Weakness in flexion and medial rotation of leg
	Superior gluteal	Tensor fasciae latae	Loss of dorsiflexion (drop foot)
	Inferior gluteal	Gluteus maximus	Limited inversion/eversion of foot
	Sciatic	Semitendinosus	Unable to extend all toes
	Sciatic	Semimembranosus	Weakness or absent plantar flexion of the foot/toes and flexion of the knee
	Deep fibular	Biceps femoris	Diminished sensation over the lateral half of the leg and the dorsum of the foot, especially the big toe and the second toe
	Deep fibular	Extensor digitorum longus	
	Deep fibular	Tibialis anterior	
	Deep fibular	Extensor hallucis longus	
	Deep fibular	Peroneus tertius	
	Deep fibular	Extensor digitorum brevis	
	Superficial fibular	Peroneus longus	
	Superficial fibular	Peroneus brevis	
	Tibial	Popliteus	
	Tibial	Tibialis posterior	
	Tibial	Flexor hallucis longus	
	Tibial	Flexor digitorum longus	

	Nerve	Muscle	Clinical findings
S1	Superior gluteal	Gluteus medius	Weakness in adduction, abduction, flexion, extension, and medial and lateral rotation of thigh
	Superior gluteal	Gluteus minimus	Weakness in flexion and medial rotation of leg
	Superior gluteal	Tensor fasciae latae	Weakness or absent plantar flexion of the foot/toes and flexion of the knee
	Inferior gluteal	Gluteus maximus	Loss of dorsiflexion (drop foot)
	Sciatic	Semitendinosus	Limited inversion/eversion of foot
	Sciatic	Semimembranosus	Unable to extend all toes
	Sciatic	Biceps femoris	Diminished sensation over the posterior, distal third of the leg, lateral heel, lateral foot, and little toe
	Deep fibular	Extensor digitorum longus	
	Deep fibular	Extensor hallucis longus	
	Deep fibular	Peroneus tertius	
	Deep fibular	Extensor digitorum brevis	
	Superficial fibular	Peroneus longus	
	Superficial fibular	Peroneus brevis	
	Tibial	Gastrocnemius	
	Tibial	Popliteus	
	Tibial	Soleus	
	Tibial	Tibialis posterior	
	Tibial	Flexor hallucis longus	
	Tibial	Flexor digitorum longus	
	Tibial	Abductor digiti minimi	
	Tibial	Quadratus plantae	
	Tibial	Flexor digiti minimi	
	Tibial	Lumbricals	
	Tibial	Adductor hallucis	
	Tibial	Abductor hallucis	
	Tibial	Flexor digitorum brevis	
	Tibial	Flexor hallucis brevis	

Continued

TABLE 7.1 ■ Upper Extremities—cont'd

Roots	Nerves	Muscles	Lower Extremities Root Lesion Signs and Symptoms
S2	Inferior gluteal	Gluteus maximus	Weakness or absent plantar flexion of the foot/toes and flexion of the knee
	Sciatic	Semitendinosus	Sensory problem over the posterior area of the leg
	Sciatic	Semimembranosus	
	Sciatic	Biceps femoris	
	Tibial	Gastrocnemius	
	Tibial	Soleus	
	Tibial	Flexor hallucis longus	
	Tibial	Flexor digitorum longus	
	Tibial	Abductor digiti minimi	
	Tibial	Quadratus plantae	
	Tibial	Flexor digiti minimi	
	Tibial	Lumbricals	
	Tibial	Dorsal interossei	
	Tibial	Plantar interossei	
	Tibial	Adductor hallucis	
	Tibial	Abductor hallucis	
	Tibial	Flexor digitorum brevis	
	Tibial	Flexor hallucis brevis	
S3	Tibial	Abductor digiti minimi	Weakness or absent plantar flexion of the foot/toes and flexion of the knee
	Tibial	Dorsal interossei	Diminished sensation over the perianal area
	Tibial	Plantar interossei	
	Tibial	Adductor hallucis	

Plexus	Nerves	Muscles	Plexus Lesion Signs and Symptoms
Lumbar plexus T12, L1–L4	Iliohypogastric	Transversus abdominis	Weakness in hip adduction and flexion
	Iliohypogastric	Internal oblique muscles	Weak or absent thigh adduction, flexion, and medial and lateral rotation
	Iliohypogastric	External oblique muscles	Weakness or inability to extend the leg at the knee
	Ilioinguinal	Transversus abdominis	Diminished sensation over the upper buttock, scrotum, or labium, hypogastric region, anterior, medial and lateral aspect of thigh, and the medial aspect of the leg
	Ilioinguinal	Internal oblique muscles	
	Genitofemoral	Cremaster	
	L1, L2, L3	Quadratus lumborum	
	L1, L2, L3	Psoas minor	
	L1, L2, L3, L4	Psoas major	
	Femoral	Iliopsoas	
	Femoral	Sartorius	
	Femoral	Rectus femoris	
	Femoral	Vastus lateralis	
	Femoral	Vastus intermedius	
	Femoral	Vastus medialis	
	Femoral	Pectineus	
	Obturator	Adductor brevis	
	Obturator	Adductor longus	
	Obturator	Gracilis	
	Obturator	Adductor magnus	
Sacral plexus L4–S3	L4, L5, S1	Quadratus femoris	Weakness in extension, adduction, flexion, and medial rotation of thigh
	L4, L5, S1	Gemellus inferior	Weakness in flexion and medial rotation of leg
	L5, S1, S2	Obturator internus	Weakness in anal sphincter
	L5, S1, S2	Gemellus superior	Diminished sensation over the posterior thigh, lateral half of the leg, and the entire foot
	S1, S2	Piriformis	
	Superior gluteal	Gluteus medius	
	Superior gluteal	Gluteus minimus	
	Superior gluteal	Tensor fasciae latae	
	Inferior gluteal	Gluteus maximus	
	Sciatic	Adductor magnus	
	Sciatic	Semitendinosus	
	Sciatic	Semimembranosus	
	Sciatic	Biceps femoris	

Continued

TABLE 7.1 ■ Upper Extremities—cont'd

Peripheral Nerves	Root	Muscles	Peripheral Nerve Lesion Signs and Symptoms
Femoral	L2, L3	Iliopsoas	Weakness in hip adduction and flexion
	L2, L3	Sartorius	Weak or absent thigh adduction, flexion, and medial rotation
	L2, L3, L4	Rectus femoris	Weakness or inability to extend the leg at the knee
	L2, L3, L4	Vastus lateralis	Diminished sensation over the anterior and medial aspect of the thigh and the medial
	L2, L3, L4	Vastus intermedius	aspect of the leg
	L2, L3, L4	Vastus medialis	
	L2, L3	Pectineus	
Obturator	L2, L3, L4	Adductor brevis	Weak or absent thigh adduction, flexion, medial and lateral rotation
	L2, L3, L4	Adductor longus	Diminished sensation over the medial aspect of the thigh
	L2, L3, L4	Gracilis	
	L2, L3, L4	Adductor magnus	
Superior gluteal	L4, L5, S1	Gluteus medius	Weakness in adduction, flexion and medial rotation of thigh
	L4, L5, S1	Gluteus minimus	
	L4, L5, S1	Tensor fasciae latae	
Inferior gluteal	L5, S1, S2	Gluteus maximus	Weakness in extension, abduction, and lateral rotation of thigh
Sciatic	L5, S1, S2	Adductor magnus	Weakness in extension of the thigh
	L5, S1, S2	Semitendinosus	Weakness in flexion and medial rotation of leg
	L5, S1, S2	Semimembranosus	Diminished sensation over the lateral half of the leg and the entire foot
	L5, S1, S2	Biceps femoris— long head	
	L5, S1, S2	Short head of biceps femoris	
Deep fibular	L5, S1	Extensor digitorum longus	Loss of dorsiflexion (drop foot)
	L4, L5	Tibialis anterior	Limited inversion/eversion of foot
	L5, S1	Extensor hallucis longus	Unable to extend all toes
	L5, S1	Peroneus tertius	Decreased sensation over the dorsum of the foot, especially the big toe and the
	L5, S1	Extensor digitorum	second toe

Nerve	Muscle	Root	Clinical findings
Superficial fibular	Peroneus longus	L5, S1	Weakness of plantar flexion
	Peroneus brevis	L5, S1	Limited eversion of foot
			Diminished sensation over the anterolateral part of the leg and the dorsum of the foot
Tibial	Gastrocnemius	S1, S2	Weakness or absent plantar flexion of the foot/toes and flexion of the knee
	Popliteus	L4, L5, S1	Inability to invert the foot
	Soleus	S1, S2	Sensory problem over the posterior area of the legs
	Tibialis posterior	L5, S1	
	Flexor hallucis longus	L5, S1, S2	
	Flexor digitorum longus	L5, S1, S2	
	Abductor digiti minimi	S1, S2, S3	
	Quadratus plantae	S1, S2	
	Flexor digiti minimi	S1, S2	
	Lumbrical	S1, S2	
	Dorsal interossei	S2, S3	
	Plantar interossei	S2, S3	
	Adductor hallucis	S1, S2, S3	
	Abductor hallucis	S1, S2	
	Flexor digitorum brevis	S1, S2	
	Flexor hallucis brevis	S1, S2	

TABLE 7.2 ■ Emg Evaluation

Muscle	Nerves	Roots
Common Upper Extremity		
Cervical paraspinal C5	Rami	C5
Cervical paraspinal C6	Rami	C6
Cervical paraspinal C7	Rami	C7
Cervical paraspinal C8	Rami	C8
Cervical paraspinal T1	Rami	T1
Deltoid	Axillary	C5–6
Biceps	Musculocutaneous	C5–6
Triceps	Radial	C6–8
Pronator teres	Median	C6–7
Abductor pollicis brevis	Median	C8–T1
First dorsal interosseous	Ulnar	C8–T1
Abductor digiti minimi	Ulnar	C8–T1
Common Lower Extremity		
Lumbar paraspinal L3	Rami	L3
Lumbar paraspinal L4	Rami	L4
Lumbar paraspinal L5	Rami	L5
Lumbar paraspinal S1	Rami	S1
Gluteus maximus	Inferior gluteal	L5–S2
Biceps femoris (short head)	Sciatic (fibular)	L5–S2
Medial gastrocnemius	Tibial	S1–2
Anterior tibialis	Deep branch of fibular	L4–5
Rectus femoris	Femoral	L2–4
Biceps femoris (long head)	Sciatic (tibial)	L5–S2
Peroneus longus	Superficial branch of fibular	L5–S1
Other Muscles Frequently Tested		
Forearm		
Flexor digitorum profundus IV and V	Ulnar	C8, T1
Flexor pollicis longus	Median (anterior interosseus)	C7–8
Flexor digitorum superficialis	Median	C7–8
Flexor carpi radialis	Median	C6–7
Flexor carpi ulnaris	Ulnar	C7–T1
Extensor indicis proprius	Radial (posterior interosseus)	C7–8
Extensor carpi ulnaris	Radial (posterior interosseus)	C7–8
Extensor carpi radialis	Radial	C6–7
Extensor digitorum communis	Radial (posterior interosseus)	C7–8
Brachioradialis	Radial	C5–6
Anconeus	Radial	C7–8
Pronator quadratus	Median (anterior interosseus)	C8, T1
Arm		
Brachialis	Musculocutaneous	C5–6
Supinator	Radial	C5–6
Extensor pollicis longus	Radial (posterior interosseus)	C7–8
Abductor pollicis longus	Radial (posterior interosseus)	C7–8
Shoulder		
Pectoralis major	Pectoral	C5–T1
Supraspinatus	Suprascapular	C5–6
Latissimus dorsi	Thoracodorsal	C6–8
Teres major	Lower subscapular	C5–6
Serratus anterior	Long thoracic	C5–7
Rhomboids	Dorsal scapular	C5
Levator scapulae	Dorsal scapular	C5
Infraspinatus	Suprascapular	C5–6
Trapezius	Spinal accessory	CN XI, C3–4

Continued

TABLE 7.2 ■ Emg Evaluation—cont'd

Muscle	Nerves	Roots
Foot		
Abductor hallucis	Medial plantar	S1–2
Abductor digiti quinti	Lateral plantar	S1–3
Leg		
Tibialis posterior	Tibial	L5, S1
Soleus	Tibial	L5–S2
Thigh		
Tensor fascia lata	Femoral	L4–5
Adductor longus	Obturator	L2–4
Vastus lateralis	Femoral	L2–4
Vastus medialis	Femoral	L2–4
Adductor magnus	Obturator, sciatic	L2–S1
Gracilis	Obturator	L2–4
Hip		
Gluteus medius	Superior gluteal	L4–S1
Iliopsoas	Femoral	L2–3
Nonlimb		
Orbicularis oris	Facial	CN VII
Orbicularis oculi	Facial	CN VII
Diaphragm	Phrenic	C3–5
Anal sphincter	Pudendal	S2–4
Sternocleidomastoid	Spinal accessory	CN XI, C2–3

This page intentionally left blank

CHAPTER 8

Pitfalls

Lyn D. Weiss

This chapter will review the physiological, technical, and human sources of error that can befall both the novice and the experienced electromyographer. Remember that if you are not getting the response that you think you should, there may be something wrong with the machine or your technique, the patient may have anomalous innervation, or you may need to rethink your diagnosis.

Pitfall 1: Poor Performance of the History and Physical Examination

Electrodiagnostic testing is an extension of your history and physical examination. Your history and physical examination are the most important components of an accurate diagnosis—not the electromyography (EMG). For example, a patient presents to you for electrodiagnostic testing with the diagnosis of carpal tunnel syndrome. On further questioning, you discover that the patient has neck pain with radiation to the hand and associated paresthesias. You suspect a cervical radiculopathy and examine the patient. The patient has a positive Spurling's test and upper extremity weakness with a decreased biceps deep-tendon reflex. Although the original consultation requested an EMG for carpal tunnel syndrome, your history and physical suggests that you should also test for a possible cervical radiculopathy. This information helps guide which nerves and muscles you will test during your EMG.

Pitfall 2: Technical Factors

Clinicians may assume that when there is an abnormal or unexpected finding, this represents pathology. However, unexpected findings may be due to an error by the electromyographer. Although technical errors are less likely in more experienced electromyographers, one reason for this is because they are acutely aware that they may need to adjust their technique if they are not getting the anticipated result. The main reason for an unobtainable or low-amplitude motor or sensory action potential (evoked response) is not stimulating the nerve and/or not recording over the appropriate nerve or muscle. This should be addressed methodically. Possible reasons for an unobtainable or low-amplitude result are:

- Is a stimulus being delivered? Look for a visible muscle contraction. If there is no muscle contraction:
  a. The stimulator is not working. Try turning down the intensity and stimulating yourself to assess whether you feel a shock.
  b. The location is incorrect. Relocate the stimulator. Or
  c. The stimulus may not be of a high-enough intensity. This may be true especially if there is excessive edema or adipose tissue. Try increasing the stimulus intensity or duration (pulse width).

■ Is the preamplifier on?

Most preamplifiers have a light indicating on/off. If the preamplifier is off, the patient will feel the shock but no response will be recorded.

■ Are the settings (gain and sweep) correct?

Attempting to elicit a sensory response with a motor setting (gain) will elicit a flat line. Sensory nerve potentials are usually about 10 to 20 μV in amplitude. Motor responses are usually in the order of 4 to 10 mV.

■ Are wires and electrodes properly connected?

A sine wave or wavy baseline usually indicates poor grounding, electrical interference, or poor electrode contact. Many machines have a notch filter that will filter out 60-Hz waves. The downside to this is that if there are any 60-Hz components to the waveform that you want, they will be filtered out as well. Changing electrodes or electrode placement may help. Sometimes unplugging electrical beds or other nonessential electrical equipment can help decrease interference.

■ Are you accurately stimulating the nerve and picking up over the muscle?

A large initial positive (downward) deflection usually indicates poor location of the electrodes or even reversal of the electrodes. Check to make sure that the reference electrode is plugged into the correct port in the preamplifier.

Is the recording electrode over the muscle from which you are trying to record? Try repositioning your recording electrode. If there is an initial positive deflection in the waveform, you may not be recording over the muscle.

Make sure that you are stimulating the nerve: look for a motor response (i.e., ankle plantarflexion when stimulating the tibial nerve).

Pitfall 3: Temperature

The temperature of the areas you are testing on your patient can affect the nerve conduction study (NCS). You should be aware that *decreasing* limb temperature could affect the latency, amplitude, conduction velocity, and duration of sensory nerve action potentials (SNAPs) and compound muscle action potentials (CMAPs) in the following manner:

■ Latency prolonged (0.2 msec/°C)
■ Amplitude increased with cooling (sensory more than motor)
■ Conduction velocity decreased (1.8 to 2.4 m/sec/°C)
■ Duration increased

You should also be aware that decreased temperature can affect the results of repetitive nerve studies and can cause normal test results in patients with neuromuscular junction disorders.

Ideally, the limb being tested should be continuously monitored for temperature by a temperature probe placed on the limb. When performing NCSs, attempt to maintain the temperature of the upper limbs above 32°C and the lower limbs above 30°C. This can be achieved by warming the area to be tested. It is always better to warm the limb rather than to use correcting formulas, as described above (i.e., correct for a temperature of 30°C in the arms by decreasing the latency by 0.4 msec). Tables 8.1 and 8.2 summarize the temperature corrections for NCSs.

Pitfall 4: Errors in Measurement

In general, the shorter the segment to be measured, the more likely an error in measurement will occur and the more dramatic will be the change in the calculated conduction velocity. For example, a 0.5-cm error in measuring distance will significantly change the conduction velocity if the measured distance is 5 cm (a 10% measurement error). However, if the distance is 10 cm and there is a

TABLE 8.1 ■ Temperature Correction for NCV Study. Expected Velocity Deviation (m/sec) From 32°C

Measured Temperature	Tibial Motor	Sural Sensory	Fibular Motor	Median Motor	Median Sensory	Ulnar Motor	Ulnar Sensory
Factor for NCV change (m/sec/°C)	1.1	1.7	2	1.5	1.4	2.1	1.6
20°C	−13.2	−20.4	−24	−18	−16.8	−25.2	−19.2
21°C	−12.1	−18.7	−22	−16.5	−15.4	−23.1	−17.6
22°C	−11	−17	−20	−15	−14	−21	−16
23°C	−9.9	−15.3	−18	−13.5	−12.6	−18.9	−14.4
24°C	−8.8	−13.6	−16	−12	−11.2	−16.8	−12.8
25°C	−7.7	−11.9	−14	−10.5	−9.8	−14.7	−11.2
26°C	−6.6	−10.2	−12	−9	−8.4	−12.6	−9.6
27°C	−5.5	−8.5	−10	−7.5	−7	−10.5	−8
28°C	−4.4	−6.8	−8	−6	−5.6	−8.4	−6.4
29°C	−3.3	−5.1	−6	−4.5	−4.2	−6.3	−4.8
30°C	−2.2	−3.4	−4	−3	−2.8	−4.2	−3.2
30.5°C	−1.65	−2.55	−3	−2.25	−2.1	−3.15	−2.4
31°C	−1.1	−1.7	−2	−1.5	−1.4	−2.1	−1.6
31.5°C	−0.55	−0.85	−1	−0.75	−0.7	−1.05	−0.8
32°C	0	0	0	0	0	0	0
32.5°C	0.55	0.85	1	0.75	0.7	1.05	0.8
33°C	1.1	1.7	2	1.5	1.4	2.1	1.6
33.5°C	1.65	2.55	3	2.25	2.1	3.15	2.4
34°C	2.2	3.4	4	3	2.8	4.2	3.2
34.5°C	2.75	4.25	5	3.75	3.5	5.25	4
35°C	3.3	5.1	6	4.5	4.2	6.3	4.8
35.5°C	3.85	5.95	7	5.25	4.9	7.35	5.6
36°C	4.4	6.8	8	6	5.6	8.4	6.4

NCV corrected = Factor × (Measured skin temperature − 32°C) − NCV measured (m/sec)
NCV, nerve conduction velocity.
From Delisa J, Lee H, Baran E, Lai K, Spielholz N. *Manual of Nerve Conduction Velocity and Clinical Neurophysiology*. 3rd ed. New York: Raven Press; 1994:17–19.

0.5-cm error in measurement, this will result in a 5% error. You should try to use segments longer than 10 cm, as there is usually some error when measuring the length of the segment.

Another source of error in measurement is not measuring over the direct course of the nerve. It is impossible to exactly measure a nerve over the skin. However, measuring over the course of the nerve will minimize the error. This is especially true of the ulnar nerve across the elbow (Fig. 8.1). The ulnar nerve is slack when the elbow is extended and taut when the elbow is bent. To measure the true length of the nerve, the elbow should be flexed to about 70 to 90 degrees both when the nerve is being stimulated and when the nerve is being measured. Measuring the nerve in the extended elbow position underestimates the true length. This will result in a calculated conduction velocity that is erroneously slow. Because all skin measurements are estimates of actual nerve length, the farther the measuring tape is from the actual nerve, the greater the potential for error. Therefore, measurements tend to be less accurate in obese patients.

Pitfall 5: Anomalous Innervation

It is important to remember that human anatomy does not always follow the textbooks and that anatomical anomalies exist. There are three anomalous innervations that are relatively common.

TABLE 8.2 ■ **Temperature Correction for Median and Ulnar Motor/Sensory Distal Latency.**
(Expected Latency Deviation From 33 Degrees C)

Measured Temperature	$-0.2\ (Tst - Tm)$[a]
20°C	−2.6
21°C	−2.4
22°C	−2.2
23°C	−2.0
24°C	−1.8
25°C	−1.6
26°C	−1.4
27°C	−1.2
28°C	−1.0
29°C	−0.8
30°C	−0.6
31°C	−0.4
32°C	−0.2
33°C	0.0
34°C	0.2
35°C	0.4
36°C	0.6

[a]$Tst = 33$°C for wrist. Tm is the measured skin temperature.
Median (or ulnar) motor or sensory NCV or distal latency corrected = $-0.2 \times (Tst - Tm)$ + Obtained NCV or distal latency
From Delisa J, Lee H, Baran E, Lai K, Spielholz N. *Manual of Nerve Conduction Velocity and Clinical Neurophysiology.* 3rd ed. New York: Raven Press; 1994:17–19.

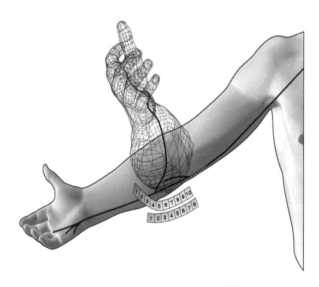

Fig. 8.1 To measure the true length of the ulnar nerve, the elbow should be flexed to about 70 to 90 degrees both when the nerve is being stimulated and when the nerve is being measured.

1. MARTIN–GRUBER ANASTOMOSIS

This is a median to ulnar nerve anastomosis in the forearm (Fig. 8.2). Nerve fibers ultimately destined for ulnar muscles travel with the median nerve and then cross over to the ulnar nerve in the forearm. These fibers then travel with the ulnar nerve into the hand and innervate ulnar muscles. They therefore do not have to traverse the carpal tunnel. This leads to three classic electrodiagnostic findings, which are more pronounced in patients with carpal tunnel syndrome.

a. Positive Deflection of CMAP

The CMAP will have an initial positive (downward) deflection when stimulating the median nerve at the elbow (but not the wrist) and when picking up over the abductor pollicis brevis (APB) muscle. The reason for this positive deflection is that ulnar fibers traveling with the median nerve stimulate the ulnar intrinsic hand muscles (specifically the adductor pollicis muscle). These fibers arrive at the adductor pollicis muscle before the median fibers arrive at the APB muscle, because they are not delayed across the carpal tunnel as the median fibers are. Because the motor point of the adductor muscle is not over the recording electrode, a positive deflection will occur.

b. Increased Conduction Velocity or Negative Conduction Velocity

The median nerve is usually slowed somewhat as it traverses the carpal tunnel. (This is why the latency for the median nerve at the wrist is usually more than the ulnar nerve at the wrist.) If a Martin–Gruber anastomosis exists, proximal median nerve stimulation will result in a *normal* latency because the fastest fibers (those upon which the latency is based) are actually ulnar fibers that do not have to travel through the carpal tunnel. The calculated conduction velocity is therefore based on a proximal stimulation (which will be falsely shortened due to the stimulation of ulnar fibers supplying the adductor pollicis muscle) and the distal stimulation (picking up over the median innervated APB muscle). With carpal tunnel syndrome, the difference in these latencies will be falsely decreased and may actually lead to a negative conduction velocity (where the elbow latency is less than the wrist latency).

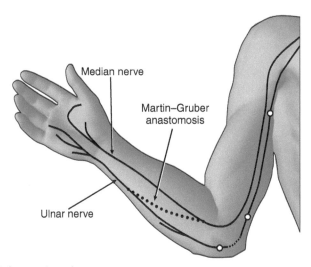

Fig. 8.2 Martin–Gruber anastomosis.

c. CMAP Amplitude Changes

With a Martin–Gruber anastomosis, the proximal CMAP amplitude will be larger than the distal amplitude (when stimulating the median nerve and picking up over the APB). This is because at the elbow, in addition to stimulating median fibers destined for the APB, ulnar fibers destined for the adductor pollicis muscle are also stimulated. Because the adductor pollicis muscle is close to the APB, the two CMAPs summate to give the appearance of a larger-amplitude CMAP with proximal stimulation. (Remember that this *larger amplitude* actually includes the response from the stimulated adductor muscle—an ulnar innervated muscle that is not usually activated with pure median nerve stimulation.) For the same reason, during ulnar motor studies, when stimulating the ulnar nerve distally (at the wrist), one may note a larger amplitude than when stimulating at the elbow. This is because some of the ulnar fibers are not being stimulated at the elbow, as they are traveling with the median nerve. The *lost* fibers in the elbow amplitude can be *found* with median stimulation at the elbow.

2. Riche–Cannieu Anastomosis

This is a communication between the deep branch of the ulnar nerve and the recurrent branch of the median nerve in the hand. With this anastomosis, the ulnar nerve may innervate the thenar muscles along with the median nerve.

If a patient with Riche–Cannieu anastomosis had a complete laceration of the median nerve at the wrist, the patient may still retain thenar muscle function, as some of these muscles may be innervated by the ulnar nerve (via the anastomosis). On EMG evaluation, a median nerve injury at the wrist, which should result in fibrillation potentials and positive sharp waves in median innervated hand muscles, may result in a normal study.

3. Accessory Fibular Nerve

The accessory deep fibular nerve (Fig. 8.3) is a branch from the superficial fibular nerve that travels posterior to the lateral malleolus and can innervate the lateral portion of the extensor digitorum brevis (EDB) muscle. Therefore a patient may have a fibular nerve injury with loss of muscle function while still maintaining EDB function. This anomaly is usually picked up when the amplitude of the fibular CMAP is larger on proximal (fibular head) stimulation than on distal (ankle) stimulation. This results because fibers from the accessory branch (posterior to the lateral malleolus) are not activated with ankle stimulation but are activated with fibular head stimulation. Usually, stimulation posterior to the lateral malleolus (with pickup over the EDB) will produce a waveform that (in amplitude) along with the ankle stimulation summates to the amplitude of the proximal (fibular head) stimulation (Fig. 8.4):

Accessory fibular nerve amplitude posterior (to lateral malleolus)
+ ankle fibular amplitude = fibular head amplitude

Pitfall 6: Stimulating Over Edematous, Subcutaneous, or Adipose Tissue

While performing NCS, be aware that stimulating over areas of edematous, increased adipose, or subcutaneous tissue can result in decreased or submaximal stimulation, as the nerve is not directly stimulated. This may result in a decreased amplitude of the CMAP. To correct this, press deeply with the stimulator until the desired results are obtained. You can also increase the pulse width. Care must be taken so as not to stimulate a different nerve located nearby. A needle may be needed for the stimulator cathode if the nerve to be tested is very deep.

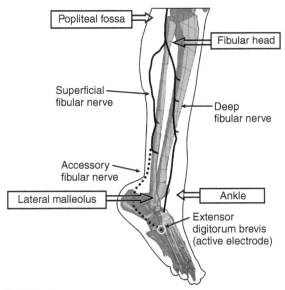

Fig. 8.3 Accessory fibular nerve.

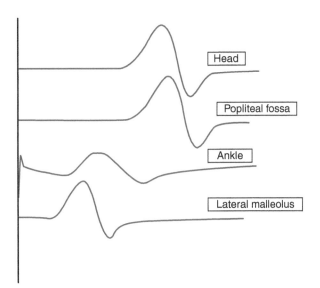

Fig. 8.4 The amplitude of the waveform produced by stimulation posterior to the lateral malleolus added to the waveform produced by stimulation at the ankle will approximate the amplitude of the waveform produced by stimulation at the fibular head. The pickup is over the extensor digitorum brevis muscle in all stimulations.

Pitfall 7: Anatomy Error

If you are stimulating or placing a needle in the incorrect nerve or muscle, obviously your results will be inaccurate. To help identify the correct muscle, have the patient activate the muscle first and palpate for correct placement. For example, to localize the APB muscle, have the patient abduct the thumb. You can then palpate the muscle as it contracts, and then you can place the electrode over the appropriate location.

Pitfall 8: Physiologic Factors

Physiologic factors can significantly affect NCS. The following factors should be considered when determining a normal or an abnormal value.

AGE

Age affects electrodiagnostic studies in both the very young and the very old patients. The effect of age is most significant from birth to 1 year when myelination is incomplete. In the newborn, nerve conduction velocities are approximately 50% of adult values.[1] By 1 year of age the velocities reach 75%; by 3 to 5 years of age, myelination is complete and children's values can be compared to adult normative data.

In adults, NCS values also change as people age. Typically, the older you get, the slower your nerves will conduct. Although these changes are fairly insignificant in the middle-aged adult, they do become more pronounced in the older adult. For example, a median motor conduction velocity of 46 m/sec in a 90-year-old patient would be normal even though generally the lower limit of normal is 50 m/sec.[1] The usual corrective factor is about 1 to 2 m/sec slowing per decade of life after age 60.[2]

In NCS, the amplitude of the SNAP and CMAP may also be affected by age. It is estimated that the SNAP amplitude may decrease by as much as 50% in a 70-year-old patient. This means that very low or even absent sensory nerve responses in the older adults should be interpreted with caution. They may be normal given the patient's advanced age. It is important to review the entire study, including the different technical factors that may affect the results, before arriving at a conclusion.

In the older adults, when dropout of motor units occurs due to normal aging, the body compensates with axonal sprouting leading to reinnervation. These reinnervated fibers are more likely to fire asynchronously. Therefore, during the EMG portion of the test in the older adult, the motor unit action potential (MUAP) duration may increase with age. In childhood, the MUAP duration increases due to physiologic growth of the muscle fiber and motor unit size.

In summary, age affects NCS in babies, with marked slowing of the velocities due to incomplete myelination. In the older adults, NCS are slower with reduced amplitudes, and normal EMG findings may include increased duration of the MUAP.

HEIGHT

Usually, the longer the extremity, the slower the distal nerves conduct. In the arms, the nerves conduct more quickly, and in shorter people they conduct more quickly. This is probably due to the fact that there is distal tapering of the nerve. The longer the limb, the more tapering and, therefore, the slower the conduction velocity will be. In addition, longer limbs are usually cooler, and this too will slow the conduction velocity. When assessing H-reflexes or F-waves, the latencies are dependent on the distances traveled. Taller people tend to have longer limbs, longer distances, and longer H-reflex and F-wave latencies.

WEIGHT

Weight is not a well-appreciated physiologic factor. However, it may be difficult to stimulate the nerve directly in obese individuals. Additional stimulus intensity or duration may be required. This is due to the electrical stimulation having to pass through additional adipose tissue before reaching the nerve. During the EMG portion of the test, technical difficulties may arise when the needle is not long enough to be easily inserted into the muscle.

Pitfall 9: Machine or Environmentally Related Nonphysiologic Factors

NOISE

Noise is any electrical signal that is not the desired biological signal you are studying. When you have a lot of noise, it is difficult to hear what you need to hear (and to see what you need to see on the screen). Electrical noise is present to some degree in all electrodiagnostic laboratories. The most frequent form of noise is 60-Hz interference, which is usually due to ubiquitous electrical appliances (e.g., lights, computers, fans, heaters). To minimize noise, check all of your equipment.

- Wires should be intact (not frayed or damaged).
- Electrodes, including the reference, should be securely attached.
- The ground should be between the recording and stimulating electrodes.
- The skin should be properly cleaned (usually with alcohol).
- Electrode gel needs to be applied.
- Sometimes wrapping the wires around each other will help reduce noise.
- Unplug equipment (e.g., examination tables) that you are not using while performing the study.
- Use the notch filter.
- Turning off fluorescent lights will cut down on the interference from unwanted signals.

Summary

- Remember to do a thorough history and physical examination.
- Know your anatomy.
- Be aware of anomalous innervations and temperature changes.
- Keep the limb appropriately warm.
- Measure correctly.
- If abnormalities are encountered, check and recheck your stimulating electrodes, wires, and placement.

References

1. Preston DC, Shapiro BE. *Electromyography and Neuromuscular Disorders*. London: Elsevier; 2012.
2. Dumitru D. *Electrodiagnostic Medicine*. Philadelphia, PA: Hanley & Belfus, Inc.; 1995:39.

CHAPTER 9

Carpal Tunnel Syndrome

Lyn D. Weiss

Carpal tunnel syndrome (symptomatic median neuropathy at the wrist) is the most common focal nerve entrapment and is a frequent reason for electrodiagnostic consultation. Electrodiagnostic testing is the best available method to assess the physiologic changes that occur in carpal tunnel syndrome.

Clinical Presentation

Classic symptoms of carpal tunnel syndrome (CTS) include paresthesias and numbness in the thumb, the index and long fingers, and the radial half of the ring finger (Fig. 9.1). Pain in the hand may also be present, and radiation proximally is not uncommon. The symptoms are frequently more prominent at night or with repetitive hand movements. The patient may complain of an inability to perform fine motor tasks and/or weakness of the hand. Certain medical and/or physical conditions predispose patients to CTS. These include diabetes, pregnancy, thyroid disorders, repetitive strain, rheumatoid arthritis, gout, peripheral neuropathy, and edema. A good history is therefore an important prerequisite to electrodiagnostic testing.

On physical examination, there may be a sensory deficit in the radial three and one-half digits. Weakness of pinch strength may also be noted. In severe cases of CTS, wasting of the thenar eminence may be present. Provocative tests may reproduce the symptoms. These include the Tinel test (percussion of the median nerve about the wrist) and the Phalen test (maximum flexion of the wrist, which is maintained for 1 to 2 minutes). Because CTS can be confused with other disorders, a thorough physical examination is always important.

Anatomy

The carpal tunnel is a fixed space that includes nine tendons (four flexor digitorum superficialis tendons, four flexor digitorum profundus tendons, and the flexor pollicis longus tendon) and the median nerve (Fig. 9.2). The carpal bones form the dorsal wall of the carpal tunnel, while the transverse carpal ligament (flexor retinaculum) provides the anterior or volar border. When the space in the tunnel becomes restricted, the median nerve can become compressed. Sensory fibers are usually affected before motor fibers.

Electrodiagnostic Findings

To do a complete electrodiagnostic assessment of the median nerve, the affected extremity must be compared to the unaffected side and to another nerve in the same hand, usually the ulnar nerve. Sensory and motor studies, as well as needle testing, should be performed. When performing nerve conduction studies (NCSs), it is imperative that the distance from the recording electrode to the stimulation site be recorded. If a person has a large hand and the distance for the distal latency for motor NCSs is not a standard distance, an increased latency will have no real meaning (Fig. 9.3). The patient's age and temperature can also contribute to changes in

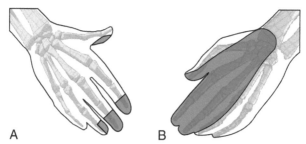

Fig. 9.1 Median nerve sensory distribution: (A) dorsal and (B) palmar.

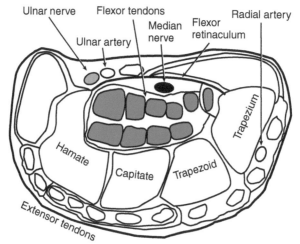

Fig. 9.2 Anatomy of the carpal tunnel.

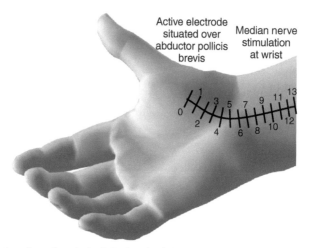

Fig. 9.3 Distance from the active electrode to the stimulation site for motor nerve conduction studies. Note that in a large hand, the distance from the abductor pollicis brevis (APB) to the wrist may be more than 8 cm. The latency will be longer if the distance is greater.

the normal latencies. It should be noted that in 10% to 15% of patients with clinical CTS, the NCSs will be normal.[1]

SENSORY NERVE CONDUCTION STUDIES

Sensory nerve action potentials (SNAPs) are usually the first potentials affected in CTS. Although antidromic or orthodromic stimulation can be used, antidromic stimulation is more common as it produces larger-amplitude SNAPs. A useful technique is to compare median SNAPs recorded at mid palm and across the carpal tunnel. Usually, a distance of 7 cm from the ring electrode on the second digit to mid palm and then another at a distance of 7 cm to the carpal tunnel (14 cm total) are used. However, because it is important to stimulate across the carpal tunnel, a larger distance can be used and recorded. Although every lab has its own standards of normal, in general a velocity of less than 44 m/sec across the carpal tunnel indicates slowing. A conduction velocity difference of greater than 10 m/sec across the carpal tunnel relative to the distal conduction velocity is also considered significant (especially because conduction velocities usually increase proximally).

Normal mid palm SNAPs confirm that the slowing is only across the carpal tunnel, although in moderate or severe cases, Wallerian degeneration may occur and affect these distal SNAPs as well. Median SNAPs may also be compared to ulnar SNAPs on the same finger. A greater than 0.5 msec difference between the two sensory latencies indicates CTS. Decreased median amplitude on the affected side could indicate either an axonal lesion of the median nerve (not specific as to where along the course of the nerve) or a conduction block across the carpal tunnel (if proximal amplitude is less than 50% of distal mid palm amplitude). An amplitude difference of more than 50% (as compared to the median sensory amplitude on the nonaffected side) is considered significant.

The combined sensory index has been used to increase diagnostic sensitivity.[2] This index combines three comparative measurements (comparing median sensory nerve slowing to ulnar and radial sensory nerves) to increase sensitivity. With a recording ring electrode over digit 4 (which is dually innervated by the median and the ulnar nerves), the median nerve is stimulated at the wrist; subsequently the ulnar nerve is stimulated at the wrist (both at 14 cm) (Fig. 9.4). An onset latency

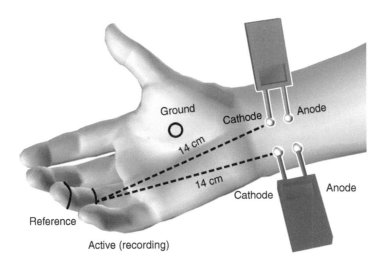

Fig. 9.4 Median to ulnar sensory latency difference. (Courtesy of Dennis Dowling.)

difference of more than 0.5 msec is considered significant. The radial and median nerves can be compared with the recording ring electrode over the thumb (as the thumb is dually innervated). The radial and median sensory nerves are stimulated at the wrist (usually at 10 cm) (Fig. 9.5). Again, a latency difference of more than 0.5 msec is considered significant. Finally, the median and ulnar mixed nerve palm latencies are compared. The nerves are stimulated orthodromically in the mid palm, and the active recording electrode is placed over the respective nerves at the wrist with a bar electrode (Fig. 9.6). A difference in latencies of more than 0.4 msec is considered significant. These three tests are then combined (latency difference in median to ulnar, latency difference in median to radial, and latency difference in median to ulnar palm). If the combined latency differences are greater than or equal to 0.9 msec, the sensitivity of diagnosing CTS is 83% with a specificity of 95%.

MOTOR NERVE CONDUCTION STUDIES

The distal latency of the compound muscle action potential (CMAP) is an important parameter in assessing for motor fiber involvement in CTS. As in sensory studies, the distance from the active electrode to the stimulation site must be standardized. Many laboratories use a distance of 8 cm. With this distance, a latency of more than 4.2 msec usually indicates CTS. The ulnar nerve must also be assessed to ensure that there is not a generalized motor neuropathy present. A median to ulnar distal latency difference of more than 1 msec also indicates CTS, as with sensory conduction studies. Decreased amplitude on the affected side could indicate either an axonal lesion of the median nerve (not specific as to where along the nerve) or a conduction block across the carpal tunnel.

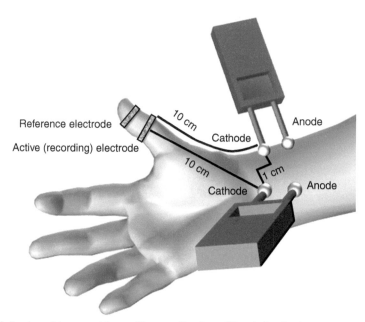

Fig. 9.5   Median to radial sensory latency difference. (Courtesy of Dennis Dowling.)

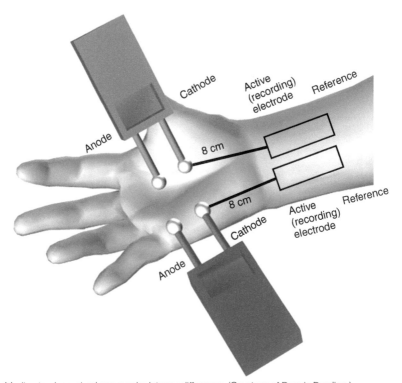

Fig. 9.6 Median to ulnar mixed nerve palm latency difference. (Courtesy of Dennis Dowling.)

LATE RESPONSES

Late responses (F-waves and H-reflexes) are generally not helpful in the evaluation of CTS because they are nonspecific and because the area of the greatest interest is not being assessed directly. The small area of slowing across the carpal tunnel is diluted by the long segment of F-waves and H-reflexes. The areas of interest are easily assessed by conventional motor and sensory studies.

ELECTROMYOGRAPHY

Electromyographic (EMG) testing should be performed to provide evidence of axonal damage (fibrillation potentials [fibs] or positive sharp waves [PSWs]) and/or reinnervation. Testing should include the abductor pollicis brevis (APB) muscle. If spontaneous activity is present in this muscle, other muscles should be tested to ensure that the diagnosis is indeed CTS, as CTS can coexist with other conditions. Specifically, a more proximal median muscle should be tested to be sure there is not a median neuropathy elsewhere along the nerve's course. In addition, a nonmedian innervated C8 muscle should be tested. Finally, especially if there is any indication of a neck problem, the cervical paraspinal muscles may be tested to rule out a cervical radiculopathy. If there is conduction block in the median nerve, recruitment may be decreased in the APB without evidence of spontaneous potentials.

TABLE 9.1 ■ Median Nerve Innervated Muscles and Expected Electromyography Changes for Focal Median Nerve Injuries

Muscles Innervated by Median Nerve From Proximal to Distal	Nerve	Muscles Affected in the Ligament of Struthers' Syndrome	Muscles Affected in Pronator Teres Syndrome	Muscles Affected in Anterior Interosseous Nerve (AIN) Syndrome	Muscles Affected in Carpal Tunnel Syndrome
Pronator teres (forearm)	Median nerve	✓	✓		
Flexor carpi radialis	Median nerve	✓	✓		
Palmaris longus	Median nerve	✓	✓		
Flexor digitorum superficialis	Median nerve	✓	✓		
Flexor digitorum profundus (digits 2 and 3)	AIN	✓	✓	✓	
Flexor pollicis longus	AIN	✓	✓	✓	
Pronator quadratus	AIN	✓	✓	✓	
Abductor pollicis brevis (distal to wrist)	Median nerve	✓	✓		✓
Opponens pollicis	Median nerve	✓	✓		✓
Flexor pollicis brevis (superficial head)	Median nerve	✓	✓		✓
First and second lumbrical	Median nerve	✓	✓		✓
Clinical sign					
Nocturnal paresthesia		Yes	Yes	No	Yes
Pain in the palm and thenar eminence		Yes	Yes, plus pain in the elbow region	No, but pain in the volar wrist or forearm	Yes
Difficult to form "O" sign		Yes	Yes	Yes	No
Weakness of pronation		Yes[a]	No	No	No
Abnormal sensation in the palm		Yes[b]	Yes[b]	No	No
NCV					
Conduction block		Upper arm to the elbow segment	Elbow to the wrist segment	No conduction block	Across the wrist

[a]Weakness of pronation differentiates ligament of Struthers' syndrome from pronator teres syndrome.
[b]The palmar cutaneous branch is spared in carpal tunnel syndrome because it passes superficial to the carpal tunnel. Sensory deficits in the palm and thenar eminence can help to differentiate pronator teres syndrome or ligament of Struthers' syndrome from carpal tunnel syndrome.

Written Report

The written conclusion should include the following:
1. Whether or not CTS is present electrodiagnostically.
2. The severity of the CTS (mild, moderate, or severe). As a general guideline:
    a. Mild—median sensory nerve conduction slowing and/or median sensory amplitude decreased but greater than 50% of reference value (no motor involvement).
    b. Moderate—Median sensory and motor slowing and/or SNAP amplitude less than 50% of the reference value.
    c. Severe—Absence of median SNAP with motor slowing or median motor slowing with decreased median motor amplitude or CMAP abnormalities with evidence of axonal injury on needle testing of the APB muscle.
3. Whether sensory and/or motor fibers are affected.
4. If spontaneous activity is noted in the APB (fibs and/or PSWs).

Summary

The classic electrodiagnostic findings in CTS may include the following:
1. Slowing of median sensory nerve conduction velocity across the carpal tunnel.
2. Prolonged distal latency of the median motor nerve.
3. Low amplitude of the median SNAP.
4. Low amplitude of the median CMAP.
5. Spontaneous potentials (fibs and/or PSWs) in the APB muscle and not in a more proximal median innervated muscle or another hand muscle innervated by C8/T1.

For a summary of NCS and EMG findings in median neuropathy, see Table 9.1.

References

1. Werner R. Electrodiagnostic evaluation of carpal tunnel syndrome and ulnar neuropathies. *PM&R.* 2013;5(suppl. 5):S14–S21.
2. Robinson LR, Micklesen P, Wang L. Strategies for analyzing nerve conduction data: superiority of a summary index over single tests. *Muscle and Nerve.* 1998;21:1166–1171.

CHAPTER 10

Ulnar Neuropathy

Lyn D. Weiss

Clinical Presentation

Ulnar neuropathy is second only to carpal tunnel as the most frequent entrapment neuropathy of the upper extremity. The ulnar nerve can be compressed at several locations along its course. Most commonly, compression occurs in its superficial location at the elbow (ulnar neuropathy at the elbow). Often this occurs when someone leans on an elbow (e.g., at a desk at work) or when the elbow is repetitively flexed and extended (e.g., a carpenter or assembly worker). Scarring of the ulnar collateral ligament, arthritis within the ulnar groove, traction at a compression site, or valgus overload in throwing athletes may each contribute to an injury. Ulnar neuropathy at the elbow can be a late effect of elbow fracture (tardy ulnar palsy). Patients typically report paresthesias, pain, and numbness in the little and ring fingers, which can worsen with elbow flexion. Pain may be experienced throughout the arm (Fig. 10.1).

Ulnar neuropathy at the wrist is less common but may occur in a canal, called Guyon's canal, formed by the hook of the hamate and the pisiform bones. These are connected by an aponeurosis, which forms the roof of Guyon's canal. This canal contains the ulnar artery, vein, and nerve. People who put a lot of pressure on their wrists, particularly in extension (e.g., cyclists and cane users) are at risk for this injury.

On physical examination in patients with ulnar neuropathy at the elbow, the ulnar nerve may be palpable in the postcondylar groove, especially with elbow flexion. There may be a sensory deficit in the fifth digit and the ulnar half of the fourth digit. Any altered sensation should be distal to the wrist, as the medial antebrachial cutaneous nerve supplies sensation above the wrist. An important clinical clue as to whether an ulnar lesion is at the elbow or the wrist is assessment of the dorsal ulnar cutaneous branch of the ulnar nerve. This nerve usually branches before the wrist, so it is spared in ulnar nerve lesions at the wrist. This nerve provides sensation to the dorsal lateral aspect of the hand. With ulnar neuropathy at either the wrist or elbow, hand intrinsic muscle weakness may be evident; and, in severe cases, clawing of the fourth and fifth digits (with attempted hand opening) and atrophy of the intrinsic muscles (particularly the first dorsal interosseous [FDI] muscle) may be obvious (Fig. 10.2).

Wartenberg's sign (abduction of the fourth and fifth digits) may occur, especially if the patient is asked to put their hands in their pants pocket. Froment's sign may also be present. This is noted when a patient is asked to grasp a piece of paper between the thumb and radial side of the second digit. When the examiner tries to pull the paper out of the patient's hand, the patient will use the flexor pollicis longus muscle (innervated by the intact median nerve) to substitute for the adductor pollicis muscle (innervated by the affected ulnar nerve) (Fig. 10.3).

On physical examination of ulnar neuropathy at the wrist, there are three basic types of lesions that can occur that affect the presentation significantly.

Type I affects the trunk of the ulnar nerve proximally in Guyon's canal and typically involves both the motor and the sensory fibers. Clinically, the patient presents with hand numbness, pain, paresthesias, and weakness in an ulnar distribution. There may be a notable sensory loss and the hand intrinsic muscles may show wasting in severe cases.

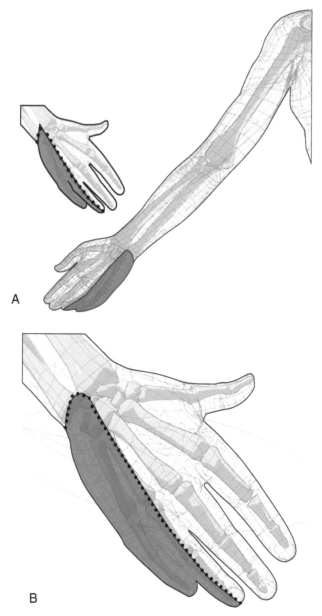

Fig. 10.1 (A) Ulnar nerve: cutaneous distribution. (B) Details of dorsum of hand.

In Type II, only the deep motor branch is affected distally in Guyon's canal. The interosseous muscles including the ulnar innervated thenar muscles are affected. Sensation is typically spared and the abductor digiti quinti (ADQ), as well as the hypothenar muscles, may or may not be spared.

In Type III, only the superficial branch of the ulnar nerve is affected. The superficial branch provides sensation to the volar aspect of the fourth and fifth fingers and the hypothenar eminence. Strength is generally preserved throughout, as is sensation of the dorsal aspect of the hand.

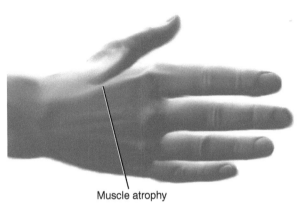

Fig. 10.2 Atrophy of the intrinsic muscles, particularly the first dorsal interosseous muscle.

Muscle atrophy

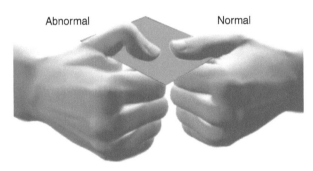

Abnormal   Normal

Fig. 10.3 Froment's sign.

Anatomy

Anatomy of the ulnar nerve renders it vulnerable to compression at two main locations: the elbow and the wrist (Fig. 10.4).

At the elbow (the most common site for ulnar nerve compression), the ulnar nerve is relatively superficial. The nerve can be compromised by pressure (such as repetitive leaning on the elbow), bony deformity (such as tardy ulnar palsy: ulnar neuropathy after a distal humeral fracture with development of a cubital valgus deformity), chronic subluxation, or in the cubital tunnel.

Cubital tunnel syndrome is compression of the ulnar nerve at or beneath the proximal edge of the flexor carpi ulnaris (FCU) aponeurosis and the arcuate ligament (also referred to as the humeroulnar arcade). With elbow flexion, the distance between the olecranon process and the medial epicondyle increases. Elbow flexion stretches and tightens the arcuate ligament, which can compress the ulnar nerve. The volume of the cubital tunnel is maximal in extension, and can decrease by 50% with elbow flexion.

The ulnar nerve is also vulnerable to compression at Guyon's canal. This is a fibro-osseous compartment in the wrist where the ulnar nerve is bound by the transverse carpal ligament, the volar carpal ligament, the pisiform bone, and the hook of the hamate. When compression occurs at Guyon's canal, the superficial and the deep branches of the ulnar nerve may be affected; however, the dorsal ulnar cutaneous nerve should be spared.

Electrodiagnostic Findings

Electrodiagnostic testing of the ulnar nerve can help to establish the existence of a lesion, to localize the injury, to prognosticate, and to exclude other conditions that may mimic an ulnar neuropathy.

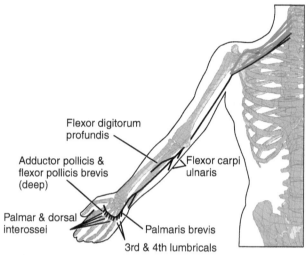

Flexor digitorum profundis

Adductor pollicis & flexor pollicis brevis (deep)

Flexor carpi ulnaris

Palmar & dorsal interossei

Palmaris brevis

3rd & 4th lumbricals

Fig. 10.4   Anatomy of the ulnar nerve.

When surgery is being considered in severe cases of ulnar neuropathy, electrodiagnostic testing can direct the surgeon to the area of entrapment. Moreover, C8 radiculopathy can present with symptoms similar to an ulnar neuropathy, and electrodiagnostic testing can help differentiate the two conditions.

While different causes of ulnar neuropathy at the elbow may benefit from different surgical procedures, electrodiagnostic studies cannot reliably and consistently differentiate between tardy ulnar palsy, retrocondylar compression, and cubital tunnel entrapment. Nevertheless, these studies can be very helpful in distinguishing ulnar neuropathy at the elbow from other pathology.

SENSORY NERVE CONDUCTION STUDIES

Sensory nerve action potentials (SNAPs) can be affected in ulnar neuropathy because the lesion is distal to the dorsal root ganglion (see Chapter 12, Radiculopathy). This is in contrast to a C8 radiculopathy, where the lesion is proximal to the dorsal root ganglion and the SNAPs are not affected. If an ulnar lesion affects the sensory fibers, SNAP amplitudes may be reduced. A side-to-side difference of more than 50% is significant for sensory axonal loss. It should be noted that a Type II lesion at the wrist, as described earlier, would affect the ulnar nerve but would spare the sensory fibers.

In an ulnar neuropathy, it is important to test not only the SNAP to the fifth digit but also the dorsal ulnar cutaneous nerve. This sensory branch of the ulnar nerve is given off 5 to 10 cm proximal to the wrist and supplies sensation to the dorsum of the fifth and ulnar side of the fourth digits. A lesion distal to the branching of the dorsal ulnar cutaneous nerve (e.g., at the wrist) should yield a normal dorsal ulnar cutaneous response, but it may show an abnormal ulnar sensory response to the fifth digit. By contrast, an ulnar neuropathy at the elbow may affect both the dorsal ulnar cutaneous response and the ulnar sensory response to the fifth digit. Because sensory responses require 50% amplitude decrement or loss of 50% of fibers to be deemed abnormal, many significant sensory lesions may not show SNAP abnormalities.

MOTOR NERVE CONDUCTION STUDIES

Slowing of latency and/or conduction velocity can indicate a demyelinating process in the ulnar nerve. In general, a prolonged distal latency of the compound muscle action potential (CMAP) indicates a slowing of the ulnar nerve across the wrist, provided there are no other indications of a generalized condition (i.e., the median distal motor latency is normal and conduction throughout the rest of the ulnar nerve is normal). Slowing of the ulnar nerve across the elbow is quite common. A conduction velocity across the elbow of less than 50 m/sec or slowing of conduction across the elbow of more than 10 m/sec (relative to the distal segment) is considered significant.[1] Similarly, a 10 m/sec velocity slowing compared to the opposite side is generally considered significant for ulnar neuropathy at the elbow.

Assessment of amplitude can be tricky, especially if a conduction block is present. Low-amplitude CMAP throughout the nerve indicates an axonal lesion. However, an amplitude drop when stimulating over a portion of a nerve indicates a conduction block (provided there is no anomalous innervation and ample stimulation is applied directly over the nerve). A drop in amplitude from the distal to the proximal site of more than 20% to 30% usually indicates either a conduction block or a Martin–Gruber anastomosis. Evaluating the median nerve CMAP morphology can check for the presence of a Martin–Gruber anastomosis (see Chapter 8, Pitfalls).

When performing nerve conduction studies of the ulnar nerve, position and measurement across the elbow are very important. The elbow should be held in a flexed position of 70 to 90 degrees. The main reasons for this are:

1. The ulnar nerve is redundant in the extended position. Therefore, measurement in extension does not measure the nerve's true anatomical length. The conduction velocity will be falsely slowed because the distance will be underestimated, and the numerator will be decreased in the equation for velocity:

$$velocity = distance/time$$

2. Maintaining the elbow in a flexed position is more likely to reproduce the symptoms of ulnar entrapment at the elbow, if it exists.

If an ulnar neuropathy is expected from the patient's clinical presentation but the ulnar CMAPs to the abductor digiti minimi (ADM) are normal, consider using the FDI muscle for the active electrode instead of the ADM. In some patients, the FDI is more affected and therefore more likely to yield a positive result.

Inching is a useful technique for localizing entrapment along the course of a nerve (Fig. 10.5). It is particularly useful in ulnar neuropathy across the elbow when surgery is being considered, as it localizes entrapment more precisely than do conventional studies. With the elbow flexed, segments of 1 cm are marked on the patient's skin both proximal and distal to the elbow. The ulnar

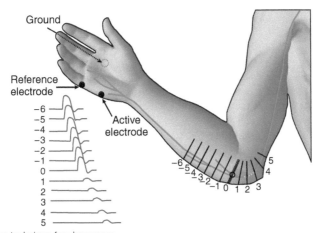

Fig. 10.5 Inching technique for ulnar nerve.

nerve is then stimulated at 1-cm intervals, and the resulting CMAPs are compared. An increase in latency of 0.4 msec/cm or greater is indicative of focal slowing. A substantial amplitude drop from one segment to a more proximal segment indicates a conduction block across that area. One must interpret these results with caution, as the margin of error is high with a small distance. Therefore, an amplitude change is much more significant than a latency change. (If more proximal stimuli, however, reveal a larger amplitude, the decreased amplitude is likely inaccurate.)

When performing nerve conduction studies across the elbow, a distance of at least 10 cm should be used to decrease the margin of error.

LATE RESPONSES

Late responses (F-waves and H-reflexes) are generally not helpful in the evaluation of an ulnar neuropathy, because they are nonspecific.

ELECTROMYOGRAPHY

Electromyographic (EMG) testing in cases of ulnar neuropathy can be difficult to interpret because of the muscles innervated by the ulnar nerve and their location. The ADM (sometimes referred to as the ADQ) and the FDI are the most commonly tested ulnar innervated hand muscles. If there is an axonotmetic lesion, these are more likely to be positive than the forearm muscles. The FDI is more likely to be involved than the ADM in deep branch or palmar lesions distal to Guyon's canal. The FCU and flexor digitorum profundus (FDP) IV and V are the only ulnar muscles proximal to the wrist. However, in ulnar nerve lesions at the elbow, the FCU and FDP muscles are usually spared. This may be to the result of:

1. the FCU and FDP receiving their innervation proximal to the medical epicondyle or
2. the fibers to the FCU being situated more laterally in the retrocondylar groove and therefore being more protected.

Consequently, if the needle examination of the FCU and FDP is negative, an ulnar nerve lesion proximal to the wrist cannot be ruled out. For this reason, the conduction studies are frequently the most important tests in localizing an ulnar lesion.

If an axonal lesion is present anywhere along the course of the nerve, spontaneous activity (fibrillation potentials [fibs] and positive sharp waves [PSWs]) may be present in muscles distal to the lesion. It is important to rule out a C8 radiculopathy by testing the cervical paraspinal muscles as well as a C8 innervated hand muscle not supplied by the ulnar nerve (i.e., the abductor pollicis brevis), which should be normal in an ulnar mononeuropathy.

Summary

In summary, the classic electrodiagnostic findings in ulnar neuropathy at the elbow may include:

1. slowing of the ulnar motor nerve conduction velocity across the elbow
2. decreased amplitude of the ulnar motor CMAP with stimulation above the elbow (conduction block)
3. decreased amplitude of the ulnar SNAP
4. spontaneous potentials (fibs and PSWs) in ulnar innervated muscles
5. decreased amplitude of the dorsal ulnar cutaneous SNAP
6. with an axonal lesion, abnormal spontaneous potentials (fibs and PSWs) may be noted in ulnar innervated hand muscles as well as the FCU. (Results should be interpreted with caution because the FCU may be negative for the reasons listed above.)

See Table 10.1 and Box 10.1 for a summary of electrodiagnostic and clinical findings in ulnar neuropathy and help to distinguish ulnar neuropathy from other conditions.

TABLE 10.1 ■ Electromyography and Clinical Findings in Focal Ulnar Nerve Injury

Location	Muscles Innervated by Ulnar Nerve From Proximal to Distal Upper Extremity and Clinical Findings	Innervated Nerve	Affected Muscles in Ulnar Entrapment Injury at Arm (Retrocondylar Groove)	Affected Muscles in Ulnar Entrapment at Elbow (Cubital Tunnel Syndrome)	Affected Muscles in Ulnar Entrapment at Wrist (Guyon's Canal)
Forearm	Flexor carpi ulnaris	Ulnar	✓	✓	
	Flexor digitorum profundus (to digits 4 and 5)	Ulnar	✓	✓	
Hand	Palmaris brevis	Ulnar	✓	✓	
	Abductor digiti minimi	Ulnar	✓	✓	✓
	Opponens digiti minimi	Ulnar	✓	✓	✓
	Flexor digiti minimi	Ulnar	✓	✓	✓
	Palmar interossei	Ulnar	✓	✓	✓
	Dorsal interossei (primarily first dorsal interosseous)	Ulnar	✓	✓	✓
	Adductor pollicis	Ulnar	✓	✓	✓
	Lumbricals (digits 4 and 5)	Ulnar	✓	✓	
Clinical sign	Paresthesia, pain, or numbness from the fourth and fifth digits and the hypothenar eminence		Up to the elbow, exacerbated by prolonged elbow flexion	Up to (or slightly distal to) the elbow, exacerbated by prolonged elbow flexion	Volar aspect only of digits 4 and 5
	Loss of sensation over the ulnar dorsal surface of the hand		Yes	Yes	No
	Claw hand		May occur	May occur	May occur
	Weakness of the flexor carpi ulnaris and the flexor digitorum profundus (digits 4 and 5)		Yes	Variable	No
	Weakness of first dorsal interosseous muscle: Froment's sign		May occur	May occur	May occur

aIn or about Guyon's canal, the ulnar nerve divides into a superficial and deep branch. The superficial branch of the ulnar nerve innervates the palmaris brevis muscle. The deep branch of the ulnar nerve travels between the abductor digiti minimi and the flexor digiti minimi muscles.

BOX 10.1 ■ Distinguishing Ulnar Neuropathy From Other Conditions

Ulnar Neuropathy at the Elbow
- Decreased sensory nerve action potential (SNAP) amplitude
- May see low-amplitude compound muscle action potentials (CMAPs) only in the ulnar nerve
- May see prolonged ulnar F-waves
- Denervation only in distal ulnar muscle
- Normal distal latency
- Decreased amplitude of dorsal ulnar cutaneous nerve

Ulnar Lesion at the Wrist
- Prolonged distal latency
- Decreased SNAP amplitude may or may not be present
- Normal dorsal ulnar cutaneous nerve

C8/T1 Radiculopathy
- Normal SNAPs
- May see low-amplitude CMAPs
- May see prolonged ulnar F-waves
- Denervation in any muscle with C8/T1 innervation, as well as paraspinal muscles

Lower Trunk Plexopathy
- Decreased SNAP amplitude
- May see low-amplitude CMAPs in ulnar and median nerves
- May see prolonged ulnar and median F-waves
- Denervation in median and ulnar muscles
- Normal paraspinals

Reference

1. American Academy of Neurology, American Association of Electrodiagnostic Medicine, American Academy of Physical Medicine and Rehabilitation. Practice parameter for electrodiagnostic studies in ulnar neuropathy at the elbow: summary statement. *Muscle Nerve.* 1999;22:408–411. Reaffirmed by the AANEM Practice Issue Review Panel: June 2015.

CHAPTER 11

Radial Neuropathy

Julie K. Silver

Clinical Presentation

As with any nerve, the radial nerve is at risk for injury in a number of locations and from a number of factors, including trauma such as a humeral fracture or compression due to an extrinsic force. The most common sites of injury are at the spiral groove (honeymooner's palsy or Saturday night palsy) and in the forearm where the nerve penetrates the supinator muscle. Less common sites include the axilla (as a result of crutches), the elbow (in radius dislocation injuries), and the wrist (as a result of handcuffs). The recurrent epicondylar branch may be associated with lateral epicondylitis or *tennis elbow*. If only the posterior interosseous branch of the radial nerve is affected, patients will complain of weakness without sensory symptoms. Injury to the antebrachial cutaneous nerve or the superficial radial sensory nerve (e.g., from lacerations at the wrist or even a watchband that is too tight) can cause numbness and paresthesias in a radial distribution (Fig. 11.1). There may or may not be associated pain. When pain is present, it can mimic or be associated with tenosynovitis (e.g., de Quervain's syndrome) of the thumb.

The physical examination is consistent with sensory and/or strength deficits that are in the distribution of the radial nerve or one of its branches. It is important to know the anatomy of the radial nerve in order to perform a competent physical examination. Usually the most obvious physical deficit is wrist drop.

Anatomy

The radial nerve branches from the posterior cord of the brachial plexus (Fig. 11.2) and in the proximal arm gives off the following sensory branches:

1. posterior cutaneous nerve of the arm,
2. lower lateral cutaneous nerve of the arm, and
3. posterior cutaneous nerve of the forearm.

Also in the proximal arm, the radial nerve supplies motor branches to the triceps and anconeus muscles. The radial nerve then wraps around the humerus in the spiral groove (one of the most common sites of injury) and supplies motor branches to the brachioradialis, the long head of the extensor carpi radialis and the supinator muscles. Just distal to the lateral epicondyle, the radial nerve splits into the posterior interosseous nerve (motor) and the superficial radial sensory nerve (sensory). The superficial radial sensory nerve supplies the lateral dorsum of the hand. The posterior interosseous nerve enters the supinator muscle under the arcade of Frohse (another common site of compression) and supplies motor nerves to the wrist, thumb, and finger extensors.

Radial nerve injuries can be classified into injuries:

- around the axilla,
- associated with the spiral groove,
- of the posterior interosseous nerve, or
- of the superficial radial sensory nerve.

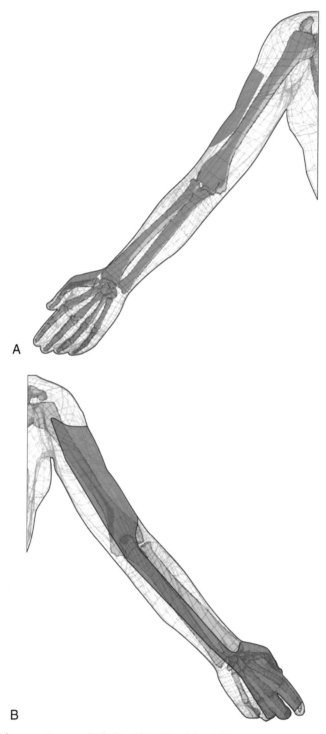

Fig. 11.1 Radial nerve, cutaneous distribution. Volar (A) and dorsal (B).

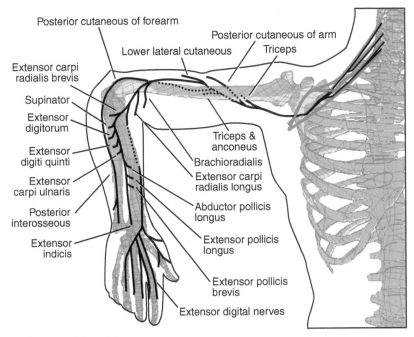

Fig. 11.2 Branches of the radial nerve.

TABLE 11.1 ■ **Common Causes of Radial Neuropathy**

Axilla	Upper Arm and Spiral Groove	Posterior Interosseous Nerve	Superficial Radial Sensory Nerve
Compression (e.g., crutches)	Compression (e.g., lateral epicondylitis, Saturday night palsy)	Compression (e.g., at the arcade of Frohse or by the supinator muscle)	Compression (e.g., handcuffs, cast, watch)
Humeral fracture (proximal) or shoulder dislocation	Humeral fracture (mid)	Radial fracture or dislocation	Trauma from intravenous line placement or iatrogenic (e.g., de Quervain injection-induced)
Benign or malignant tumor	Benign or malignant tumor	Benign or malignant tumor	Benign or malignant tumor

The radial nerve is responsible for the so-called Saturday night palsy which is classically compression of the radial nerve when someone who perhaps is very fatigued or intoxicated lies with the arm draped over the back of a chair or some other fixed object. However, there are a variety of reasons why the radial nerve may be injured (Table 11.1).

Electrodiagnostic Findings

SENSORY NERVE CONDUCTION STUDIES

If the superficial radial sensory nerve is affected, in demyelinating lesions there may be a prolonged distal latency or, in the case of conduction block (neurapraxia), decreased or unobtainable response if the lesion is distal to the site of stimulation. In axonal lesions there will be reduced amplitude of the sensory nerve action potential (SNAP) regardless of the location of the lesion (as long as it is distal to the dorsal root ganglion). In cases where the SNAP is normal but the patient clinically has a radial sensory deficit, this may be because the study was done too early (it takes 4 to 7 days for Wallerian degeneration to occur); because the lesion may be proximal to the dorsal root ganglion (i.e., root level); or because a demyelinating lesion (causing either focal slowing or conduction block) may be proximal to the site of stimulation.

MOTOR NERVE CONDUCTION STUDIES

Radial motor studies can be very helpful in diagnosing radial nerve injuries. In axonal injuries, there is a reduction in the compound muscle action potential (CMAP) amplitude after 4 to 7 days. This can be compared to the contralateral (unaffected) side. Radial conduction velocities may appear to be abnormally fast (e.g., more than 75 m/sec), but the value of doing this study is to look for a focal conduction block or decreased amplitude. In primarily demyelinating lesions at the spiral groove, the CMAPs recorded at the elbow, forearm, and below can be normal; however, stimulation proximal to the spiral groove (across the lesion) may reveal marked temporal dispersion or a decrease of amplitude or area (evidence of conduction block).

LATE RESPONSES

Late responses are nonspecific and not typically done in suspected radial neuropathy.

ELECTROMYOGRAPHY

The electromyography (EMG) will typically be abnormal in motor axonal radial nerve lesions. It may demonstrate the usual findings seen in an axonal neuropathy (e.g., spontaneous activity, large motor unit action potentials with long duration, and possibly polyphasic in chronic cases). Because the extensor indicis muscle is the most distal muscle innervated by the radial nerve, it is often tested first. If abnormal, more proximal radial innervated muscles should be tested. Through needle EMG the radial nerve can be *mapped out* distal to proximal until normal radial innervated muscles are reached. The crux of the EMG study in a radial neuropathy is to locate the lesion by knowing the anatomy (see Fig. 11.2).

Tables 11.2 and 11.3 are a summary of nerve conduction studies (NCSs)/EMG and clinical findings in radial neuropathy. A muscle innervated by C7, but not by the radial nerve (such as the pronator teres or flexor carpi radialis muscle), should be tested. Such muscles would be normal in a radial nerve injury, but may be abnormal in a C7 radiculopathy. If the radial nerve injury is in the axilla, the triceps muscle may be abnormal, but the deltoid muscle (innervated by the axillary nerve) should be normal. It should also be noted that in patients with a supinator syndrome, the supinator muscle itself would be normal. This is because the radial nerve innervation to the supinator muscle branches proximally to the muscle itself. The radial nerve is compressed in the supinator muscle after the supinator has received its innervation.

Summary

In summary, electrodiagnostic findings in radial neuropathy may include the following (depending on the location and type of lesion):
1. Decreased amplitude of the radial SNAP
2. Decreased amplitude of radial CMAP
3. Slowing of radial motor conduction velocity across the affected segment (or increased distal latency)

TABLE 11.2 ■ **EMG and Clinical Findings in Focal Radial Nerve Injury**

Location	Muscles Innervated by Radial Nerve From Proximal to Distal Upper Extremity and Clinical Signs	Nerve	Muscles Showing Neurogenic Change in the Crutch Palsy (Posterior Cord Injury) and Clinical Findings	Muscles Showing Neurogenic Change in the Saturday Night Palsy (Spiral Groove Injury) and Clinical Findings	Muscles Showing Neurogenic Change in Posterior Interosseous Nerve Syndrome and Clinical Findings
Shoulder	Deltoid[a]	Axillary[a]	Yes		
	Triceps	Radial	Yes	Yes	
Arm	Anconeus	Radial	Yes	Yes	
Forearm	Brachioradialis	Radial	Yes	Yes	
	Extensor carpi radialis	Radial	Yes	Yes	
	Supinator	PIN[b]	Yes	Yes	Yes
	Extensor carpi ulnaris	PIN[b]	Yes	Yes	Yes
	Extensor digitorum communis	PIN[b]	Yes	Yes	Yes
	Extensor digiti minimi	PIN[b]	Yes	Yes	Yes
	Abductor pollicis longus	PIN[b]	Yes	Yes	Yes
	Extensor pollicis longus	PIN[b]	Yes	Yes	Yes
	Extensor pollicis brevis	PIN[b]	Yes	Yes	Yes
	Extensor indicis	PIN[b]	Yes	Yes	Yes
Clinical signs	Decreased distal radial sensation		Yes	Yes	No
	Weakness of abduction of shoulder		Yes	No	No
	Weakness of extension of shoulder		Yes	No	No
	Weakness of extension of elbow		Yes	Yes	No
	Weakness of extension of wrist		Yes	Yes	Depends on the location of lesion
	Weakness of extension of MCP		Yes	Yes	Yes
	Weakness of DIP/PIP extension		Yes	Yes	Yes
	Weakness of supination of forearm		Yes	Yes	Depends on the location of the lesion

[a]The deltoid, while not radially innervated, is innervated by the axillary nerve, which arises from the posterior cord with the radial nerve.
[b]PIN is a motor branch of the radial nerve.
DIP, Distal interphalangeal; *EMG*, electromyography; *MCP*, metacarpophalangeal; *PIN*, posterior interosseous nerve; *PIP*, proximal interphalangeal.

TABLE 11.3 ▪ NCS/EMG and Clinical Findings in Radial Neuropathy

Radial Nerve Entrapment Location	Nerve Involved	Is Sensory Affected?	Muscles Affected
Axilla	Radial and axillary	Yes	All radial muscles plus deltoid
Spiral Groove	Radial	Yes	Anconeus and distal (triceps spared)
Superficial radial sensory	Superficial radial sensory	Yes	None
Posterior interosseous	PIN	No	Supinator and distal (supinator spared in supinator syndrome)

EMG, Electromyography; *NCS*, nerve conduction study; *PIN*, posterior interosseous nerve.

4. A drop in radial CMAP amplitude only across the affected segment (conduction block)
5. Spontaneous potentials (fibrillation potentials and positive sharp waves in radially innervated muscles distal to lesion)
6. Recruitment abnormalities
7. If the posterior interosseous nerve (a motor branch) is affected, the radial CMAP may be abnormal, but the radial SNAP should be normal. (This may be seen in the supinator syndrome.)
8. If the superficial radial sensory nerve (a pure sensory nerve) is affected, the radial SNAP may be abnormal, but the radial CMAP should be normal.

CHAPTER 12

Radiculopathy

Lyn D. Weiss

Radiculopathy is a lesion of a specific nerve root and is generally caused by root compression. It is second only to carpal tunnel syndrome (CTS) as the reason for referral for electrodiagnostic study. The diagnosis of radiculopathy is based on a patient's history, physical examination, and electrodiagnostic study. Electrodiagnostic testing should never be performed without a thorough history and physical, which is used to guide the examination. Imaging studies are complementary. The diagnosis of radiculopathy is contingent upon motor and sensory symptoms and/or findings in a distribution consistent with a nerve root. In certain clear-cut clinical scenarios, electrodiagnosis may not be necessary.

Often, however, in the case of a radiculopathy or possible radiculopathy, electrodiagnostic studies are quite helpful in making or confirming the diagnosis and in determining the prognosis. Although magnetic resonance imaging (MRI) may be helpful in anatomically localizing a lesion, it does not give physiological information. In one study of asymptomatic patients, 27% had disk protrusions on MRI.[1] On the other hand, although an electromyogram (EMG) does not reveal the anatomy in the same way that imaging studies do, it provides physiological information about the nerves and muscles. In addition, electrodiagnostic testing can exclude conditions that may mimic radiculopathy, such as mononeuropathies, plexopathies, or polyneuropathies. Therefore, both imaging studies (usually an MRI) and electrodiagnostic studies are extremely helpful in confirming the diagnosis of a radiculopathy.

Clinical Presentation

Patients with radiculopathy will frequently complain of neck pain radiating to the arm (cervical radiculopathy) or back pain radiating to the leg (lumbosacral radiculopathy). The patient may also complain of numbness or tingling in the distribution of a sensory nerve root, referred to as a dermatomal distribution (see Fig. 18.2). Thoracic radiculopathies, while rare (less than 2% of radiculopathies), would radiate pain and/or numbness in the distribution of the nerve root. In addition, if the motor fibers are affected, there will be weakness of muscles innervated by that nerve root, referred to as a myotomal distribution (Tables 12.1 and 12.2). For example, a patient with a right L5 radiculopathy may complain of back pain radiating to the right leg, numbness along the lateral aspect of the right leg into the dorsum of the foot, and foot slap with walking. Radiculopathies typically affect one extremity. Symmetrical weakness is unlikely to be due to a radiculopathy; if findings are symmetrical, an alternate diagnosis should be sought.

On physical examination, the patient with a right L5 radiculopathy may have normal reflexes, decreased sensation on the lateral aspect of the right leg and dorsum of the right foot, and weakness of the ankle dorsiflexors. It is important to remember that not all patients experience the same symptoms. In addition, dermatomal and myotomal distributions may vary among individuals. It is possible for a radiculopathy to affect predominantly sensory fibers, motor fibers, or both. Physical findings that may suggest a radiculopathy include the following:

- decreased reflexes (e.g., a decreased ankle reflex in an S1 radiculopathy),

TABLE 12.1 ■ Clinical Picture—Cervical Radiculopathy[2]

Root Level	Muscle Group	Clinical Sign
C5	Rhomboid (dorsal scapular nerve) Supraspinatus/infraspinatus (supra-scapular nerve) Deltoid/teres minor (axillary nerve) Biceps brachii/brachialis (musculocutaneous nerve)	Positive neck distraction/compression test Decreased/absent biceps tendon reflex Decreased/absent sensation to the lateral arm (axillary nerve) Weakness of shoulder abduction
C6	Extensor carpi radialis longus and brevis (radial nerve) Pronator teres/flexor carpi radialis (median nerve) Deltoid/teres minor (axillary nerve)	Decreased/absent brachioradialis reflex Decreased/absent sensation to the lateral forearm (musculocutaneous nerve) Weakness of wrist extension
C7	Triceps/extensor digitorum communis/extensor indicis proprius digiti minimi (radial nerve) Flexor carpi radialis (median nerve) Flexor carpi ulnaris (ulnar nerve)	Decreased/absent triceps reflex Decreased/absent sensation to the middle finger Weakness of wrist flexion
C8	Flexor carpi ulnaris (ulnar nerve) Flexor pollicis longus/flexor digitorum superficialis (median nerve) Flexor digitorum profundus (median or ulnar nerve) Extensor indicis proprius/extensor pollicis brevis (radial nerve) First dorsal interosseous (ulnar nerve)	Decreased/absent sensation to the ring and little fingers of the hand and to the distal half of the forearm's ulnar side (ulnar nerve) Weakness of finger flexion Intrinsic weakness and atrophy
T1	Abductor pollicis brevis (median nerve) Abductor digiti minimi/dorsal interosseous (ulnar nerve)	Decreased/absent sensation to medial side of the upper half of the forearm and the arm (medial brachial cutaneous nerve) Weakness of finger abduction/adduction

- weakness in muscles innervated by that nerve root (because most muscles are innervated by multiple nerve roots, this may not be apparent), and
- sensory symptoms in a dermatomal distribution.

The physical examination has several limitations that may make electromyography (EMG) a necessary adjunct in the diagnosis of radiculopathy. A mild weakness can be missed easily on manual muscle testing. If the patient is stronger than the examiner, subtle weakness in the upper extremities may not be apparent. The examination is not quantitative, and a loss of 10 pounds of biceps strength, for example, may be imperceptible. Lower extremity muscles such as the quadriceps can exert forces greater than the total body weight, and only severe weakness will be apparent. In many cases of clinically missed weakness, EMG will be positive. For instance, a 10% loss of motor axons may reveal no perceptible weakness on physical examination; however, EMG testing is likely to be sensitive enough to detect the abnormality.

Anatomy

Electrodiagnostic evaluation of a radiculopathy requires a thorough knowledge of the anatomy of the spine. There are 31 pairs of spinal nerves attached to the spinal cord by ventral and dorsal roots.

TABLE 12.2 ■ Clinical Picture—Lumbosacral Radiculopathy[2]

Root Level	Muscles	Clinical Sign
L2, L3, L4[a]	Iliacus/vastus medialis (femoral nerve) L2–L3	Pain in the thigh
	Adductor longus/gracilis (obturator nerve) L2–L4	Weakness in hip flexion, adduction
L4	Vastus lateralis, rectus femoris	Decreased/absent patellar reflex[b]
	Tibialis anterior (deep fibular nerve) L4–L5	Pain in the medial side of the leg
	Vastus medialis and lateralis (L2–L4)	Knee extension weakness
L5	Gluteus medius/tensor fasciae latae (superior gluteal nerve L4–S2, posterior)	Pain and paresthesias in the lateral aspect of the leg and the dorsum of the foot
	Flexor hallucis longus/flexor digitorum longus/lateral gastrocnemius/tibialis posterior (tibial nerve, L5–S2)/tibialis anterior	Ankle dorsiflexor weakness
	Extensor hallucis longus/extensor digitorum longus (deep fibular nerve, L5)	
S1[c]	Medial gastrocnemius/soleus/flexor hallucis brevis (tibial nerve, L5–S2)	Decreased/absent ankle reflex
	Peroneus longus and brevis (superficial fibular nerve, L5, S1)/tensor fascia lata/gluteus maximus (superior/inferior gluteal nerve L4–S1/L5–S2)	Pain and paresthesias to the lateral border of the foot
	Extensor hallucis longus, extensor digitorum (deep fibular nerve, L4–S1)	Weakness of foot plantar flexion and toe extension

[a]Lesions of L2, L3, and L4 are best considered collectively because they have such extensive myotomal overlap. Consequently, it is frequently impossible to distinguish isolated lesions involving one of them. It can be difficult to diagnose an L2 or an L3 radiculopathy. The L2–L3 myotomes have limited limb representation. All the muscles innervated by the L2–L3 myotomes are located proximally in the lower extremity, and they are reinnervated sooner than muscles located more distally. There is no reliable sensory nerve conduction study available for evaluating the L2–L4 fibers. In L4 radiculopathies, similar changes may be found in the tibialis anterior muscle, but their absence cannot exclude a lesion of that root.
[b]The patellar reflex is a deep-tendon reflex, mediated through nerves emanating from the L2, L3, and L4 nerve roots, but predominantly from L4. For clinical application, the patellar reflex is considered an L4 reflex; however, even if the L4 nerve root is totally cut, the reflex can still be present in significantly diminished form.
[c]H-reflex may assist in the diagnosis and helps to distinguish S1 from L5 radiculopathy.

The spinal nerve is a mixed sensory and motor nerve that is formed by the fusion of ventral and dorsal roots in the intervertebral foramina (see Fig. 1.1).
■ The ventral roots are axons with cell bodies in the anterior horn cells in the ventral gray matter of the spinal cord. These roots are from motor neurons whose axons terminate in a neuromuscular junction.
■ The dorsal roots are axons with cell bodies in the dorsal root ganglia in the vertebral foramina, outside the spinal cord. These are sensory axons.
The cell body of sensory fibers is outside the spinal cord, as opposed to motor fibers where the cell body is within the spinal cord. In a radiculopathy, there is usually continuity between the

sensory cell body and the digits, because the lesion is proximal to the dorsal root ganglia. Although sensation may be altered, electrodiagnostically the sensory nerve action potential (SNAP) will not be affected (see Fig. 1.1).

All of the muscles that are innervated by a single ventral root define a myotome. A dermatome is the sensory distribution of a single nerve root. Except for the rhomboid muscle, which is predominantly innervated by the C5 root, almost every muscle is innervated by multiple roots and is therefore part of multiple myotomes. When performing a physical examination, it should be kept in mind that dermatomes (the skin area innervated by a single dorsal root) also overlap.

Electrodiagnostic Medicine Evaluation
SENSORY NERVE CONDUCTION STUDIES

Pain, numbness, and tingling are common complaints in patients with radiculopathy. However, in the majority of radicular processes, the SNAP should be normal, both in amplitude and latency. Latency is contingent on the speed of the fastest fibers. Amplitude is contingent on the number of fibers firing. Damage to the myelin sheath of an axon would generally cause slowing or conduction block. This would be apparent on nerve studies if the lesion were between the area of stimulation and the recording electrodes.

In radiculopathy, any demyelination is proximal to the area being stimulated, and therefore conduction block or slowing will not be seen. Basically this means that *sensory nerve conduction studies (NCSs) should be normal* unless there is alternate or coexisting pathology (e.g., CTS). When there is axonal damage and the distal parts of the axon are no longer contiguous with the cell body, the axon will die back, a process known as Wallerian degeneration. In a radiculopathy, any damage to the dorsal (sensory) fibers is generally proximal to the dorsal root ganglion. Therefore as the axon is still in contact with its cell body, no sensory denervation will occur. Even in severe lesions that result in anesthesia, normal sensory studies are usually noted. If SNAP abnormalities are found, it is important to rule out other lesions distal to the dorsal root ganglion, such as a brachial plexopathy, an entrapment neuropathy, or a peripheral neuropathy. It should be noted that in a radiculopathy affecting only sensory fibers, the electrodiagnostic study should be normal.

MOTOR NERVE CONDUCTION STUDIES

Compound muscle action potential (CMAP) amplitudes reflect the actual number of motor fibers activated upon stimulation. The latency is a function of the speed of the fastest distal fibers. In general, both the sensory and motor NCS will be normal in an isolated case of radiculopathy. However, in a severe radicular lesion (which is distal to the anterior horn cell), axonal loss can result in Wallerian degeneration distal to the lesion. Therefore the CMAP amplitude may be affected (reduced).

Nonetheless, even with a lesion that causes axonal degeneration, the CMAP amplitude could still be normal. This is because the muscles have input from multiple nerve roots and motor units. The radicular lesion may impinge on nerve fibers that do not innervate the muscle being tested, or fibers from other nerve roots may contribute more significantly and therefore the amplitude will not be significantly affected. For example, if the C8 nerve root is affected, the amplitude of a CMAP recorded from the abductor pollicis brevis (APB) muscle is usually not affected. In addition to receiving fibers from C8, the APB receives innervation from T1. There would have to be a complete (or near complete) lesion of either C8 or T1 to see a significant decrease in amplitude compared to the nonaffected side. Because the lesion is proximal to the area being stimulated, no slowing or conduction block should be present on motor nerve studies.

From these discussions, it should be apparent that motor and sensory studies are of limited use in radiculopathies. When abnormalities occur they are likely to be of motor nerve (CMAP) amplitude. Increased distal latencies, slowing or conduction block, or decreased SNAP amplitude would suggest an alternate diagnosis. In fact, the main value of NCSs in testing for radiculopathy is to rule out other diagnoses, such as a peripheral or entrapment neuropathy.

LATE RESPONSES

The H-reflex is a monosynaptic or oligosynaptic spinal reflex involving both motor and sensory fibers. It electrically tests some of the same fibers as are tested in the ankle jerk reflexes. In fact, it is rare to be unable to obtain an H-reflex in the presence of an ankle jerk reflex. If this occurs, technical factors should be considered. In theory, it is a sensitive measure in assessing radiculopathy because it helps to assess proximal lesions, it becomes abnormal relatively early in the development of radiculopathy, and it incorporates sensory fiber function proximal to the dorsal root ganglion. The H-reflex primarily assesses afferent and efferent S1 fibers. Clinically, L5 and S1 radiculopathies may appear similar on EMG due to the overlap of myotomes. The H-reflex's primary value is in distinguishing S1 from L5 radiculopathies.

When assessing for S1 radiculopathy, the H-reflex latency is recorded from the gastrocnemius–soleus muscle group upon stimulating the tibial nerve in the popliteal fossa (Fig. 12.1). The H-reflex is elicited with a submaximal stimulation with the cathode proximal to the anode. As the stimulation is gradually increased from peak H-amplitude, we generally see a diminishment of the H-amplitude with a concurrent increase in the M-wave amplitude. With supramaximal stimulation, the H-reflex is usually absent.

Although the H-reflex is sensitive, it is not specific and has certain limitations. First, patients with an S1 radiculopathy can have a normal H-reflex. Second, an abnormal H-reflex is only suggestive, but not definitive, for radiculopathy because the abnormality may originate in other components of the long pathway involved, such as the peripheral nerves, plexuses, or spinal cord. Third, once the H-reflex becomes abnormal, it usually does not return to normal, even over time. Finally, the H-reflex is often absent in otherwise normal individuals over the age of 60 years. The reflexes therefore can be considered a sensitive, but not specific, indicator of pathology. Latency of

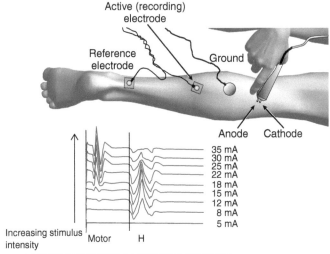

Fig. 12.1 Assessment for S1 radiculopathy by performing an H-reflex.

the H-reflex is dependent on the age and leg length of the patient (see Table 4.1). A side-to-side amplitude (comparing the results obtained from one leg to the results of the other leg) difference of 60% or more may also indicate pathology. Generally, gastrocnemius–soleus H-reflex latency side-to-side differences of greater than 1.5 msec are suggestive of S1 radiculopathy.

The H-reflex can also be obtained in the upper extremity by recording over the flexor carpi radialis (FCR) muscle and stimulating the median nerve at the elbow. The clinical utility of the FCR H-reflex for cervical radiculopathies (C6 or C7) has yet to be established.

F-waves are low-amplitude, late responses thought to be due to antidromic activation of motor neurons (anterior horn cells) following peripheral nerve stimulation, which then cause orthodromic impulses to pass back along the involved motor axons. Some electromyographers have called this a *backfiring* of axons. It is called the F-wave because it was first noted in intrinsic foot muscles. The F-wave has a small amplitude, a variable configuration, and a variable latency. Generally, F-wave amplitudes are on the order of 1% of the orthodromically generated motor response (M-response). The F-wave can be found in many muscles of the upper and lower extremities. Unfortunately F-waves are not sensitive tests. The reasons for this are as follows:

1. The pathways involve only the motor fibers.
2. As with the H-reflex, the F-wave involves a long neuronal pathway so that a focal lesion would likely be obscured.
3. If an abnormality is present, the F-wave will not pinpoint the exact cause because any lesion, from the anterior horn cell to the muscle being tested, can affect the F-wave similarly.
4. Because muscles have multiple root innervations, the shortest latency may reflect the healthy fibers in the nonaffected root.
5. The latency and amplitude of an F-wave are variable so that multiple stimulations must be performed to find the shortest latency.

F-waves are neither sensitive nor specific. F-waves are not useful in the evaluation of radiculopathy.[3] See Table 4.2 for a comparison of H-reflex and F-waves.

ELECTROMYOGRAPHY

EMG is the most useful diagnostic study in localizing radiculopathy and predicting prognosis. In cases of radiculopathy causing axonal damage, Wallerian degeneration will occur. Muscle fibers supplied by these axons will begin to fire spontaneously. This spontaneous activity in the form of fibrillation potentials (fibs) and/or positive sharp waves (PSWs) initially occurs in proximal muscles and extends distally with time. These potentials have a characteristic appearance and sound.

The presence of spontaneous activity is the most objective evidence of acute denervation. Lesser lesions may cause increased insertional activity, although the subjective nature in determining these lowers the confidence level in diagnosis. In reinnervation and with sprouting of collateral axons, motor unit action potential abnormalities such as high amplitude, long duration, or polyphasic motor units may be noted in affected muscles. Recruitment abnormalities, if seen, would be typical of a neuropathic recruitment including few motor units firing at a high rate (higher than 20 Hz), as described in Chapter 5, Electromyography.

Spontaneous activity as seen by EMG begins in the proximal paraspinal muscles, usually within 5 to 7 days of compression. Most limb muscles show spontaneous activity within 3 weeks, but 5 to 6 weeks may be required in the distal portions of the limb. Similarly, reinnervation usually occurs in a proximal-to-distal manner. One should keep in mind that the needle EMG will be able to assess only axonal injury to motor fibers.

The selection of muscles to be tested is of critical importance. The needle examination should be sufficiently detailed to distinguish between lesions at the root, plexus, and peripheral nerve level. Paraspinal muscles are useful to indicate a root level lesion, as opposed to more peripheral etiologies. However, due to overlapping innervation of the paraspinal muscles, a specific level

TABLE 12.3 ■ Levels of Confidence in Diagnosis of Cervical or Lumbosacral Radiculopathy

EMG Diagnosis	Mildly Suggestive	Moderately Suggestive	Strongly Suggestive/ Definitive
Muscles with neurogenic change	Early change in paraspinals or one root innervated muscle without motor/sensory NCS change	Early change in paraspinals and two or more same root innervated muscles without motor/sensory NCS change Acute denervation and/ or chronic change on paraspinals and any one spinal root innervated muscle	Acute denervation and/ or chronic change in two muscles from two different peripheral nerves but same myotome, as well as paraspinal involvement

EMG, Electromyography; NCS, nerve conduction study.

cannot be determined without corresponding abnormalities in limb muscles. The muscles noted to be weak on examination, or muscles with abnormal tendon reflexes, should be examined to maximize the yield of the study. In fact, the physical examination serves as the foundation upon which the electrodiagnostic study is performed. Without an adequate history and physical examination, the yield of the electrodiagnostic studies is significantly lowered. There is not enough time, and it would be unkind to your patient to attempt to examine every possible muscle. Therefore the study needs to be tailored to fit the specific clinical circumstances.

To have a definitive diagnosis of radiculopathy, a paraspinal muscle and two muscles from different peripheral nerves innervated by the same root should have positive findings. If only some (but not all) of the criteria are met, the diagnosis of radiculopathy is only suggestive (Table 12.3). It is also important to note that if the patient has only sensory involvement, the NCS/EMG test may be completely normal. Remember that the SNAP will not be affected, and the EMG assesses only motor fibers. In these cases the EMG may be performed to rule out other causes for the patient's symptoms. The report should specify that, while the study is normal, radiculopathy cannot be ruled out, and it may be appropriate to refer for other diagnostic tests.

Summary

In summary, electrodiagnostic findings in radiculopathy may include:
1. normal SNAP amplitude and conduction velocity,
2. normal CMAP latency, amplitude and conduction velocity (predominantly), and
3. spontaneous potentials (fibs and PSWs) in the paraspinal muscles and two muscles from different peripheral nerves innervated by the same affected root level.

Tables 12.2 and 12.3 provide summaries of clinical findings in radiculopathy.

References

1. Jensen MC, Brant-Zawadzki MD, Obuchowski N, Modic MT, Malkasian D, Ross JS. Magnetic resonance imaging of the lumbar spine in people without back pain. *N Engl J Med.* 1994;331:69–73.
2. Wilbourn AJ. AAEM minimonograph #32: the electrodiagnostic examination in patients with radiculopathies. *Muscle Nerve.* 1998;21:1612–1631.
3. Lin C-H, Tsai Y-H, Chang C-H, et al. The comparison of multiple F-wave variable studies and magnetic resonance imaging examinations in the assessment of cervical radiculopathy. *Am J Phys Med Rehabil.* 2013;92(9):737–745.

CHAPTER 13

Spinal Stenosis

Lyn D. Weiss

Spinal stenosis can be defined as a narrowing or restriction of the vertebral canal and can affect any spinal level. The spinal cord, cauda equina, and/or nerve root structures may be involved.

Clinical Presentation

Patients with spinal stenosis usually complain of back or neck pain with radiation to one or both extremities. Patients with lumbar stenosis usually complain of a dull ache in the hip and thigh region. The pain is typically relieved with sitting, which tends to flex the spine and therefore increase the diameter of the spinal canal. This is referred to as *neurogenic claudication*. (In true vascular claudication, the patient only has to stop walking and rest to relieve the symptoms, not necessarily flex the spine.)

Anatomy

The spinal canal usually has an anteroposterior diameter of at least 13 mm. A canal diameter of 10 to 13 mm is considered a relative stenosis and less than 10 mm is an absolute stenosis.[1]

The condition may be due to congenital or acquired factors. These factors can include spondylolisthesis, enlargement of the soft tissues in and around the canal, hypertrophy of the facet joints, intervertebral disk herniation, or ligamentum flavum hypertrophy or laxity.

Electrodiagnostic Findings

Although electrodiagnostic testing in spinal stenosis may be nonspecific, testing is helpful to rule out other causes for the patient's symptoms, including radiculopathy, peripheral neuropathy, or entrapment neuropathy. It is important to note that electrodiagnostic studies are not typically performed as means of diagnosing spinal stenosis. This diagnosis is usually made on the basis of history, physical examination, and imaging studies.

SENSORY NERVE CONDUCTION STUDIES

Sensory nerve conduction studies (NCSs) and amplitudes should be *normal* in spinal stenosis. This is due to the fact that the sensory (dorsal) root ganglion is located outside the spinal canal and therefore is usually not affected in spinal stenosis.

MOTOR NERVE CONDUCTION STUDIES

Motor NCSs should demonstrate normal distal latencies, as the distal aspect of the nerve is not affected. Compound muscle action potential (CMAP) velocities and amplitudes are usually unaffected, unless the disease has progressed to the point that there is significant axonal damage and motor axon collateral sprouting cannot keep pace with axonal damage. In such cases, one may see decreased amplitude of the CMAP on NCSs.

LATE RESPONSES

H-reflexes may be prolonged or absent bilaterally if the S1 nerve root is affected by the spinal stenosis. F-waves are generally not helpful in the evaluation of spinal stenosis because they are nonspecific.

ELECTROMYOGRAPHY

If neural compression is significant, multilevel bilateral needle abnormalities may be noted, including fibrillations and positive sharp waves (in acute neural compression). With chronic neural compression, the motor unit action potentials may be of large amplitude, polyphasic, and of increased duration. It is important to test multiple bilateral paraspinal levels and multiple myotomal levels in both extremities.

Summary

Similar to radiculopathies, sensory and motor NCSs are typically normal with the exception of severe axonal loss, in which case one may note decreased amplitude of the CMAP.

The classic electrodiagnostic findings in spinal stenosis may include:

1. Normal sensory nerve action potential amplitudes and conduction velocities
2. Normal CMAP latency, amplitude, and conduction velocities
3. EMG findings of bilateral multilevel root involvement.

Reference

1. Isaac Z, Lopez E. Lumbar spinal stenosis. In: Frontera W, Silver J, Rizzo T, eds. *Essentials of Physical Medicine and Rehabilitation*. 3rd ed. Philadelphia: Elsevier; 2015:257–263.

CHAPTER 14

Fibular (Peroneal) Neuropathy

Julie K. Silver

Clinical Presentation

Fibular neuropathy is the most common mononeuropathy in the legs and occurs due to compression, entrapment, ischemia, or direct trauma. The fibular nerve has traditionally been called the peroneal nerve because another name for the fibula is perone. However, recent revisions in anatomic terminology have encouraged the use of the term *fibular nerve*. This can also help to prevent confusion with a similar sounding nerve, the perineal nerve.

The most likely site of compression of the fibular nerve is at the fibular neck (or head), where the nerve is very superficial (Fig. 14.1). The patient typically presents with foot drop that is usually acute but may be gradual. There may be a history of recent falls or tripping as well. Paresthesias and numbness in the lower lateral leg and dorsum of the foot may be present. Pain is typically absent.

A thorough history can help determine the cause of the symptoms (e.g., a plaster cast that was too tight, a habit of crossing the legs, a brace that doesn't fit well, occupational squatting as a carpenter would do). Fibular neuropathy can easily be confused with lumbar radiculopathy (usually L5), sciatic neuropathy, or lumbosacral plexopathy. Electrodiagnostic studies can be crucial to determining the location and extent of damage.

In fibular neuropathy, both the deep and superficial fibular nerves are usually affected. In cases where only one branch is affected, deep fibular neuropathy is more common than superficial fibular neuropathy. The examination findings will vary depending on the affected nerve(s) (Fig. 14.2). Because the deep fibular nerve provides sensation to the first dorsal web space, assessment of sensory deficits in this region can help localize the lesion. Strength deficits are usually most notable in ankle dorsiflexion and great toe extension. There may be a foot slap or steppage gait when the patient ambulates. Reflexes are typically normal. Tinel's sign may be present over the fibular neck.

Anatomy

The common fibular nerve arises from the L4 to S1 nerve roots that travel through the lumbosacral plexus and then through the sciatic nerve. Within the sciatic nerve, the fibers that eventually form the common fibular nerve run separately from those that distally become the tibial nerve (separation of these nerves usually occurs just above the popliteal fossa).

The fibular division of the sciatic nerve innervates the short head of the biceps femoris. This is important electrodiagnostically as it is the only muscle proximal to the knee that is innervated by the fibular nerve. In fibular neuropathy at the fibular neck, the short head of the biceps femoris muscle should not be affected.

The common fibular nerve gives off a sensory branch supplying the lateral surface of the knee (the lateral cutaneous nerve of the knee) and then winds around the fibular neck and passes through the *fibular tunnel* between the peroneus longus muscle and the fibula. It then divides into superficial and deep branches. The superficial fibular nerve innervates the peroneus longus and brevis muscles and terminates in sensory branches that supply the lateral aspect of the lower leg and the dorsum of the foot and toes. In 15% to 25% of people, the superficial fibular nerve also

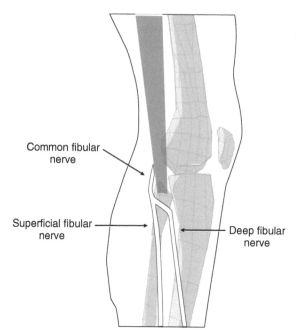

Fig. 14.1   Fibular nerve.

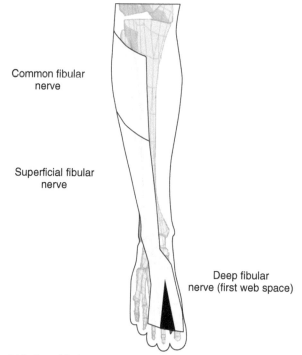

Fig. 14.2   Sensory distribution of fibular nerve.

gives rise to the *accessory fibular nerve*. This provides an anomalous innervation of the extensor digitorum brevis (EDB) (see Chapter 8, Pitfalls).

The deep fibular nerve (also called the anterior tibial nerve) supplies the tibialis anterior (TA), extensor digitorum longus, extensor hallucis longus, peroneus tertius, and EDB muscles. The terminal sensory branches supply the skin over the first dorsal web space.

Electrodiagnostic Findings

SENSORY NERVE CONDUCTION STUDIES

The superficial sensory fibular nerve study is not significantly more technically demanding than the sural sensory study; however, it is often not done. Nevertheless, when there is a question of a fibular neuropathy, it is an important study to perform. In lesions that are axonal or mixed axonal and demyelinating, the superficial fibular sensory nerve action potential (SNAP) amplitude can be low or absent. However, in purely demyelinating lesions at the fibular neck, the distal superficial fibular sensory response remains normal.

MOTOR NERVE CONDUCTION STUDIES

In demyelinating lesions, focal slowing or conduction block can be noted in fibular motor studies across the fibular neck. Proximal slowing of more than 10 m/sec compared to the distal conduction velocity indicates focal slowing. A drop in amplitude of the proximal fibular compound muscle action potential (CMAP) (compared to distally) of more than 20% suggests conduction block.

If axonal loss is predominantly present, then fibular CMAP amplitudes will be reduced at all stimulation sites (e.g., ankle, below the fibular head and lateral popliteal fossa) because the pickup is over a distal muscle whose nerve supply has undergone Wallerian degeneration (the EDB muscle). The motor nerve conduction velocity and the distal latency may be slightly slowed or normal, depending on whether the fastest conducting axons have been lost. Often there is a combination of demyelination and axonal loss in the same patient.

The EDB is usually the site of recording for motor studies. However, it is not unusual for the EDB to be atrophied for nonpathologic reasons (e.g., as the result of wearing tight shoes). Therefore, although the EDB is the usual site of recording, it may be worthwhile to consider recording over the TA muscle. If you do the study over the EDB and it does not show focal slowing or conduction block, then consider repeating the study using the active electrode over the TA, which may pick up the deficit. Of course, if there is any question of an abnormal study, you can compare it to the contralateral side as well.

If the proximal amplitude to the EDB is greater than the distal amplitude, an accessory fibular nerve should be considered. A stimulation posterior to the lateral malleolus will yield a CMAP at the EDB in this case (see Chapter 8, Pitfalls).

LATE RESPONSES

In fibular neuropathy at the fibular neck, F-wave responses may be prolonged or absent on the affected side and normal on the unaffected side. If fibular F-waves are performed with ankle stimulation, the slowing may be more pronounced than with popliteal stimulation, as the F-response crosses the area of slowing two times with ankle stimulation and only once with fibular or popliteal stimulation. It must be remembered, however, that these responses are nonspecific and should not be used to diagnose fibular neuropathy. H-reflexes are usually done to rule out an alternate diagnosis and should be normal in fibular neuropathy because they do not involve the fibular nerve.

TABLE 14.1 ■ Muscle Involvement in Focal Fibular Nerve Injury

Location	Muscles Innervated by Fibular Nerve From Proximal to Distal Lower Extremity	Nerve	Neurogenic Change in Muscles in Fibular Nerve Injury Above Fibular Head/Sciatic Nerve Injury in Buttock	Neurogenic Change in Muscles in Fibular Nerve Injury to the Fibular Head	Neurogenic Change in Muscles in Deep Fibular Neuropathy	Neurogenic Change in Muscles in the Superficial Fibular Neuropathy
Thigh	Biceps femoris (short head)	SN-F	✓			
Leg	Extensor digitorum longus	DF	✓	✓	✓	
	Tibialis anterior	DF	✓	✓	✓	
	Extensor hallucis longus	DF	✓	✓	✓	
	Peroneus tertius	DF	✓	✓	✓	
	Extensor digitorum brevis	DF	✓	✓	✓	
	Peroneus longus	SF	✓	✓		✓
	Peroneus brevis	SF	✓	✓		✓
Clinical sign	Foot drop, weakness of foot dorsiflexion, high-stepping gait		Yes	Yes	Yes	No
	Weakness of foot eversion		Yes	Yes	No	Yes
	Pain, loss of sensation, or numbness		Anterolateral part of the leg up to lateral side of the popliteal fossa and/or the dorsum of the foot[a]	Anterolateral part of the leg and the dorsum of the foot[b]	A small area between the first and second toes[c]	Most of the foot's dorsum except the region between the first and second toes[b]
	Tinel's sign may be present		No	Fibular head	No	No

[a]Lateral cutaneous nerve of the calf.
[b]Lateral and medial terminal branches of SF nerve.
[c]Terminal branches of DF nerve.

DF, Deep fibular nerve; SF, superficial fibular nerve; SN-F, sciatic nerve, fibular division.
Adapted from Leis AA. Atlas of Electromyography. Oxford University Press; 2000:135–145.
Dumitru D, Amato AA, Zwarts M, eds. Electrodiagnostic Medicine. 2nd ed. Hanley & Belfus; 2002:898–905.

ELECTROMYOGRAPHY

Needle electromyography (EMG) testing is abnormal in axonal fibular lesions when significant axonotmesis is present. Abnormalities will be found in fibular-innervated muscles distal to the lesion. In axonal lesions, there will be evidence of spontaneous activity, positive sharp waves and fibrillation potentials, and decreased recruitment of motor unit action potentials (MUAPs). In chronic axonal lesions, there may be evidence of decreased recruitment of MUAPs, and the morphology of the MUAPs may be long duration, high amplitude, and polyphasic. In predominantly demyelinating lesions, only decreased MUAP recruitment (with normal firing frequency) will occur, and the MUAP morphology will be normal. The EMG is important to rule out other nerve lesions. Therefore proximal leg and paraspinal muscles are often tested (to rule out a radiculopathy), and tibial-innervated muscles are sampled below the knee. It is important to note that the tibial nerve supplies the hamstring muscles, with the exception of the fibular innervated short head of the biceps femoris muscle.

The short head of the biceps femoris can be very helpful in distinguishing a fibular nerve injury at the fibular head from a sciatic nerve injury affecting predominantly fibular fibers. Due to the anatomy of the sciatic nerve (as noted earlier), the fibular fibers can be more susceptible to injury than the tibial (especially in the sciatic notch and buttock region). In instances where insults could have occurred to the buttock region and the fibular head (i.e., trauma, foot drop after hip surgery), the short head of the biceps femoris may be the main distinguishing factor between these lesions.

Summary

The classic electrodiagnostic findings in a fibular neuropathy at the fibular neck may include:
1. Reduced fibular CMAP amplitude compared to the contralateral side
2. Fibular motor nerve conduction block or focal slowing across the fibular neck
3. Reduced superficial fibular SNAP amplitude
4. Absent or prolonged fibular F-response on the affected side
5. Normal sural sensory, tibial motor, and H-reflexes
6. EMG findings of spontaneous activity and/or reinnervation in muscles supplied by the deep and superficial fibular nerves
7. Normal EMG findings in the short head of the biceps femoris, paraspinal muscles, and tibially innervated muscles

See Table 14.1 for a summary of electrodiagnostic findings in fibular neuropathy.

CHAPTER 15

Tarsal Tunnel Syndrome

Julie K. Silver   ■   Jay M. Weiss

Clinical Presentation

Classic or proximal tarsal tunnel syndrome (TTS) involves an entrapment neuropathy of the entire tibial nerve behind the medial malleolus under the flexor retinaculum or laciniate ligament, whereas distal TTS involves a terminal branch (or branches) of the tibial nerve. In distal TTS, the most commonly involved nerve is the lateral plantar, but the medial plantar and medial calcaneal branches are also frequently involved.

TTS is much less common than other neuropathies such as carpal tunnel syndrome or fibular neuropathy and is often more difficult to diagnose. This neuropathy is nearly always unilateral. Conditions that may lead to TTS include trauma, space-occupying lesions, biomechanical problems causing joint deformity, and systemic diseases. Some cases are idiopathic as well.

Patients with TTS generally complain of pain around the ankle (especially on the medial side) that may be elicited or exacerbated by manual palpation, and/or paresthesias typically accompanied by numbness over the sole of the foot. Weakness in the foot is not very common in this neuropathy. TTS can be an overlooked cause of heel pain as the inferior calcaneal nerve (first branch of the lateral plantar nerve) supplies anterior calcaneal sensation before innervating the abductor digiti minimi.

On physical examination there may be a positive Tinel's sign over the tibial nerve at the medial ankle (Fig. 15.1). The sensory examination might be abnormal over the plantar surface of the foot. Subtle weakness is not well appreciated because it is often difficult to isolate the muscles supplied by the involved nerve(s).

Anatomy

TTS involves entrapment of the tibial nerve or any of its branches in the region beneath the flexor retinaculum at the medial ankle. In addition to the tibial nerve, the tibial artery and tendons of the flexor hallucis longus, flexor digitorum longus, and tibialis posterior muscles pass through the tarsal tunnel (Fig. 15.2). While there is some variability, there are generally four terminal branches of the tibial nerve.

The medial calcaneal nerve branches off proximal in (or above) the tarsal tunnel and is a purely sensory branch supplying sensation to the medial ankle and heel. The remaining nerve then gives off the medial and lateral plantar nerves. The first branch of the lateral plantar nerve (also called the inferior calcaneal nerve or in some literature Baxter's nerve) supplies sensation to the anterior calcaneus and innervates the abductor digiti minimi.

Both plantar nerves innervate the intrinsic muscles of the foot. The medial plantar nerve typically supplies the first three toes and the medial half of the fourth toe, while the lateral plantar nerve supplies the lateral fourth toe and the entire fifth toe. It is useful to think of the medial and lateral plantar nerves as the median and ulnar nerves of the foot. The medial plantar nerve is analogous to the median nerve, which also generally supplies sensation to the first three and one-half digits, while the lateral supplies the last one and one-half digits (again similar to the ulnar nerve in

147

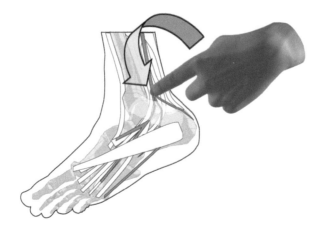

Fig. 15.1 Tinel's sign over the tibial nerve.

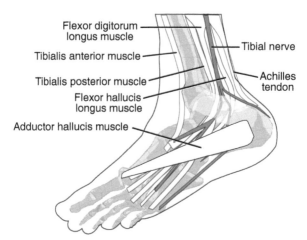

Fig. 15.2 Anatomy of the tibial nerve.

the hand). Carrying this analogy further, the medial plantar branch supplies the abductor hallucis, while most of the foot intrinsics (including interossei) are innervated by the lateral plantar nerve.

Electrodiagnostic Findings

SENSORY NERVE CONDUCTION STUDIES

In TTS, the medial and lateral plantar sensory nerve action potential (SNAP) may be affected or absent. However, this should be interpreted with caution because pure SNAPs are difficult to obtain in the foot and frequently require averaging. Also, the foot is very sensitive to temperature changes. It is important to note that medial and lateral plantar sensory nerves are often hard to obtain even in normal patients. In general, pure sensory studies have limited usefulness in TTS and are replaced by mixed nerve studies.

TABLE 15.1 ■ Electromyography and Clinical Findings in Focal Tibial Nerve Injury

Location	Muscles Innervated by the Tibial Nerve and Clinical Findings	Nerve Involved	Neurogenic Changes in Tibial Nerve Injury Above the Knee and Clinical Findings	Neurogenic Change on Muscles in the Tarsal Tunnel Syndrome and Clinical Findings[a]
Leg	Gastrocnemius	Tibial nerve	✓	
	Popliteus	Tibial nerve	✓	
	Soleus	Tibial nerve	✓	
	Tibialis posterior	Tibial nerve	✓	
	Flexor hallucis longus	Tibial nerve	✓	
	Flexor digitorum longus	Tibial nerve	✓	
Foot	Abductor digiti minimi	Lateral plantar nerve	✓	✓
	Quadratus plantae	Lateral plantar nerve	✓	✓
	Flexor digiti minimi	Lateral plantar nerve	✓	✓
	Dorsal interossei	Lateral plantar nerve	✓	✓
	Plantar interossei	Lateral plantar nerve	✓	✓
	Adductor hallucis	Lateral plantar nerve	✓	✓
	Lumbrical	Medial plantar nerve	✓	✓
	Abductor hallucis	Medial plantar nerve	✓	✓
	Flexor digitorum brevis	Medial plantar nerve	✓	✓
Clinical sign	Nocturnal paresthesias		Variable	Common
	Burning in the sole of the foot		Variable	Common
	Tinel's sign over the tarsal tunnel		No	Common
	Inability of plantar flexion		Variable	No
	Decreased sensation in plantar aspect of the foot		Common	Common

[a]Tarsal tunnel syndrome is caused by compression of the tibial nerve or its branches at the tarsal tunnel.

MOTOR NERVE CONDUCTION STUDIES

These, along with mixed nerve studies, are the most common and important studies done in TTS. The distal latency of the medial plantar nerve (to the abductor hallucis) or the lateral plantar nerve (to the abductor digiti minimi), or both, may be increased in TTS if demyelination is present. Because motor latencies are less temperature sensitive than sensory latencies, you can compare medial and lateral latencies and compare both latencies to the contralateral (unaffected) side. If axonal loss is prominent, then the compound muscle action potential will be reduced and the distal latencies will be normal or just slightly prolonged.

Motor nerve studies for TTS should include assessing both the medial and lateral plantar branches. Only studying the tibial nerve to the abductor hallucis is analogous to only studying the median nerve in the hand to exclude a possible ulnar lesion.

MIXED NERVE CONDUCTION STUDIES

Mixed nerve studies are typically performed orthodromically (with regards to the sensory fibers) and require stimulation on the plantar surface and surface pickup over the tibial nerve posterior to the medial malleolus. These are small responses and should be obtained on the unaffected side before attempting on the involved side. Both medial and lateral plantar mixed nerve studies should be performed as part of a TTS study.

The use of mixed nerve studies increases the sensitivity of electrodiagnostic studies for TTS.

LATE RESPONSES

F-waves may be abnormal but are nonspecific and not typically done in TTS studies. H-reflexes should be normal in TTS.

ELECTROMYOGRAPHY

Electromyography (EMG) of the foot is usually quite difficult, in part because patients tolerate this exam poorly (due to pain). Additionally, many patients have difficulty isolating specific muscles for activation. There is a debate in the medical literature as to whether there can be evidence of spontaneous activity as well as long duration and large amplitude motor unit action potentials in foot muscles in healthy people without nerve injuries. Some authors consider the needle EMG of foot muscles (both medial and lateral plantar innervated) to be a very important part of the electrodiagnostic evaluation for TTS. It is recommended that you perform an EMG in tibial innervated muscles both above and below the level of the tarsal tunnel and that you check fibular (peroneal) innervated muscles as part of the differential diagnosis. If a positive finding is noted, consider checking the unaffected foot to rule out the possibility of a normal variant.

Summary

In summary, electrodiagnostic findings in TTS may include:
1. prolonged or low amplitude of the medial and/or lateral plantar mixed nerves responses,
2. prolonged distal latency of the medial or lateral plantar motor nerve,
3. decreased amplitude of the medial or lateral plantar motor nerve, and
4. spontaneous potentials (fibrillation potentials and positive sharp waves) in muscles innervated by the medial or lateral plantar nerve.

See Table 15.1 for a summary of nerve conduction study (NCS)/EMG findings in TTS.

CHAPTER 16

Peripheral Polyneuropathy

Lyn D. Weiss

Peripheral neuropathies are generalized dysfunctions of nerves. They represent a collection of disorders with the commonality of damage to the nerves in the peripheral nervous system. Electrodiagnostic testing can determine if a peripheral polyneuropathy exists, how severe it is, and its characteristics. Based on the characteristics of the neuropathy (e.g., axonal, demyelinating, sensory, motor) the electromyographer can direct the referring clinician toward a suspected cause (or causes) for the neuropathy (Table 16.1).

Clinical Presentation

Symptoms of peripheral polyneuropathy usually begin in the feet with numbness, pain, and/or paresthesias. As the disease progresses, patients may report that they feel weaker or that they are tripping more frequently. When the hands are affected, activities of daily living (ADLs) may be affected. It is important to note that regardless of strength, loss of sensation will markedly affect function, making it difficult to walk, button a shirt, make a phone call, write a letter, or perform other ADLs. Peripheral neuropathies are commonly seen in people with diabetes and individuals who drink alcohol excessively. There are many other medical conditions that are associated with peripheral polyneuropathy as well. A good history should include asking about symptoms in family members, because some neuropathies are hereditary.

On physical examination, the patient may have findings consistent with the specific type of neuropathy. For example, a patient with a motor axonal neuropathy may have weakness in the distal muscles with decreased deep tendon reflexes. Patients with a predominantly sensory neuropathy may have diminished sensation to light touch, pinprick, temperature, and vibration. If the feet and hands are predominantly affected, the patient is referred to as having a *stocking–glove* distribution of symptoms.

Anatomy

Peripheral neuropathies are classified as affecting primarily motor fibers, sensory fibers, or both. They are also classified as to what part of the nerve is predominantly affected: axon, myelin, or both (Fig. 16.1). Finally, neuropathies are classified as segmental (affecting only certain areas of the nerve) or uniform (affecting the entire length of the nerve). Most neuropathies affect the distal segment of the nerve more than the proximal segment. Therefore the longer the nerve, the more it is usually affected. This explains the predominance of findings in the feet in patients with neuropathy.

Standard nerve conduction tests do not test autonomic or small fibers, which may be affected in a peripheral polyneuropathy.

TABLE 16.1 ■ Polyneuropathy

EMG Finding	Uniform Demyelinating Mixed Sensorimotor Polyneuropathy	Segmental Demyelinating Motor > Sensory Polyneuropathy	Axon Loss Motor > Sensory Polyneuropathy	Sensory Axon Loss Neuropathy	Axon Loss Mixed Sensorimotor Polyneuropathy	Mixed Axonal Loss and Demyelinating Sensorimotor Polyneuropathy
CMAP amplitude	Normal	Decreased secondary to dispersion or conduction block	Decreased	Normal	Decreased	Decreased
Motor latency	Increased	Increased	Normal	Normal	Normal	Increased
Motor conduction velocity	Decreased	Decreased	Normal	Normal	Normal	Decreased
Dispersion of CMAP	No	Yes	No	No	No	No
SNAP amplitude	Normal	Normal or decreased	Decreased (usually)	Decreased	Decreased	Decreased
SNAP conduction velocity	Decreased	Decreased (somewhat)	Normal	Normal	Normal	Decreased
Needle EMG: Would fibs and PSWs likely be noted?	No (normal)	No (normal)	Yes	No (normal). Needle EMG assesses motor fibers only.	Yes	Yes

Common diseases					
1. Hereditary motor sensory neuropathy type I, III, VI (distal weakness with little atrophy) 2. Metachromatic leukodystrophy 3. Krabbe's leukodystrophy 4. Adrenomyeloneuropathy 5. Congenital hypomyelinating neuropathy 6. Tangier disease 7. Cockayne's syndrome 8. Cerebrotendinous xanthomatosis	1. AIDP: Guillain–Barré syndrome (ascending proximal weakness) 2. CIDP (weakness of asymmetric low extremities) 3. Osteosclerotic myeloma 4. Leprosy 5. Acute arsenic polyneuropathy 6. Pharmaceuticals (amiodarone perhexiline) high-dose Ara-C carcinoma, AIDS	1. Paraneoplastic motor neuronopathy (distal weakness) 2. Porphyria 3. Axonal Guillain–Barré syndrome 4. Hereditary motor sensory neuropathy types II and V 5. Lead neuropathy 6. Dapsone neuropathy	1. Paraneoplastic (sensory, painful in distal extremities) 2. Hereditary sensory neuropathy types I–IV 3. Friedreich's ataxia 4. Spinocerebellar degeneration 5. Abetalipoproteinemia (Bassen–Kornzweig disease) 6. Primary biliary cirrhosis 7. Acute sensory neuronopathy 8. Cisplatin toxicity 9. Lymphomatous sensory neuronopathy Chronic idiopathic ataxic neuropathy 10. Sjögren's syndrome 11. Fisher variant Guillain–Barré syndrome 12. Paraproteinemias 13. Pyridoxine toxicity 14. Amyloidosis	1. Alcoholic polyneuropathy (distal symmetric weakness) 2. Vitamin (thiamine, B12) deficiency (distal symmetric weakness) 3. Gouty neuropathy 4. Metal neuropathy (e.g., mercury, thallium, gold) 5. Sarcoidosis 6. Connective tissue diseases (e.g., rheumatoid arthritis, SLE) 7. Gastrectomy, gastric restriction surgery for obesity 8. Chronic liver disease 9. Neuropathy of chronic illness 10. Hypothyroidism 11. Myotonic dystrophy 12. AIDS 13. Critical illness neuropathy 14. Lyme disease 15. Vincristine neuropathy 16. Toxic neuropathy (acrylamide, carbon disulfide, carbon monoxide)	1. Diabetic polyneuropathy (distal symmetric weakness) 2. Uremia (distal symmetric weakness)

AIDP, Acute inflammatory demyelinating polyneuropathy; *CIDP*, chronic inflammatory demyelinating polyneuropathy; *CMAP*, compound muscle action potential; *EMG*, electromyography; *fibs*, fibrillation potentials; *PSWs*, positive sharp waves; *SLE*, systemic lupus erythematosus; *SNAP*, sensory nerve action potential.

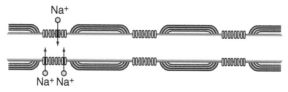

Normal axon and distribution of myelin

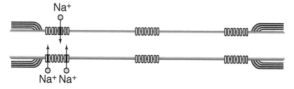

Injury to myelin
Note: A demyelinated axon does not become an unmyelinated axon

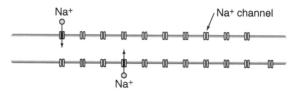

Unmyelinated axon
Note: Uniform distribution of sodium (Na⁺) channels in
unmyelinated axon compared to demyelinated axon

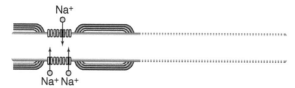

Injury to axon

Fig. 16.1   Characteristics of nerve injury.

Electrodiagnostic Findings

To adequately assess for a peripheral polyneuropathy, sensory and motor nerves must be tested in at least three extremities. Because temperature can affect latency, amplitude, and conduction velocity (see Chapter 8, Pitfalls), limb temperature should be maintained at 32°C for the upper extremities and 30°C for the lower extremities. Table 16.1 will help you identify the type of neuropathy based on the electrodiagnostic findings.

SENSORY NERVE CONDUCTION STUDIES

If a peripheral polyneuropathy involves the sensory fibers, sensory nerve action potentials (SNAPs) may be affected. If the sensory neuropathy is axonal in nature, the amplitude of the SNAP will be affected, or the response may be unobtainable. If the sensory neuropathy is demyelinating, the SNAP responses can have a decreased conduction velocity. A profound demyelinating process or a distal conduction block can also result in the loss of SNAPs.

MOTOR NERVE CONDUCTION STUDIES

If a peripheral polyneuropathy involves motor fibers, the compound muscle action potential (CMAP) may be affected. If the motor neuropathy is axonal in nature, the amplitude of the CMAP may be affected, or it may be unobtainable. If the motor neuropathy is demyelinating, the CMAP response may have an increased distal latency and/or slowed conduction velocity. Conduction velocity less than 80% of the lower limit of normal suggests a demyelinating neuropathy. A conduction block can result in the diminution or loss of CMAP amplitude if the nerve is stimulated proximal to the conduction block.

It should be noted whether conduction velocity slowing is uniform throughout the nerve (uniform demyelination) or whether it only affects certain segments of the nerve (segmental demyelination). In segmental demyelination, some of the fibers are traveling slower than other fibers. The CMAP that is generated will be dispersed, meaning it will have a longer duration and lower amplitude (temporal dispersion) (see Fig. 6.1). In general, inherited (congenital) demyelinating polyneuropathies are usually uniform. Temporal dispersion generally implies an acquired rather than a congenital neuropathy.

LATE RESPONSES

Because late responses (F-waves and H-reflexes) assess the peripheral nerve along its entire course, these responses are usually affected in peripheral polyneuropathy. In diseases such as Guillain–Barré syndrome, F-waves can be the earliest indications of a problem, because the proximal segment of the nerve is tested. It should be remembered, however, that these responses are not specific. Therefore, the information generated can help, but not confirm, the diagnosis.

ELECTROMYOGRAPHY

Electromyography (EMG) findings are usually negative in peripheral polyneuropathy, unless a severe axonal motor neuropathy is present. In such cases, affected muscles may demonstrate spontaneous activity (fibrillation potentials and positive sharp waves) in distal muscles. Complex repetitive discharges may be noted in chronic neurogenic disorders. Both proximal and distal muscles should be tested. EMG testing is helpful, even when negative, because it helps rule out other disorders, such as a focal neuropathy or myopathy. In addition, if an axonal lesion is present, the severity as well as the time course of the disease can be assessed (see Chapter 5, Electromyography).

Summary

In summary, electrodiagnostic findings in peripheral polyneuropathy may include:
1. Increased latency and/or decreased conduction velocity in demyelinating neuropathies (increased motor latency and/or decreased conduction velocity in motor demyelinating neuropathies and increased sensory latency and/or decreased conduction velocity in sensory demyelinating neuropathies).
2. Decreased amplitude of the CMAP or SNAP in axonal neuropathies (decreased CMAP amplitude in motor axonal neuropathies and decreased SNAP amplitudes in sensory axonal neuropathies).
3. Abnormal spontaneous activity may be found on needle study in motor axonal neuropathies.

See Table 16.1 for a summary of nerve conduction study (NCS)/EMG findings in peripheral polyneuropathy.

CHAPTER 17

Myopathy

Julie K. Silver

Clinical Presentation

A myopathy is simply a disorder of the muscles. This can take various forms; the common myopathic disorders are listed in Table 17.1. The primary symptom in myopathy is *weakness*. It is important to note that most myopathies affect the *proximal* muscles more than the distal muscles. This means that the first symptom a patient may complain about is difficulty rising from a chair or walking up stairs.

The weakness is *constant* but may be more noticeable when someone is fatigued. In conditions where distal weakness is more prominent (e.g., hereditary distal myopathies), patients may complain of foot drop, unstable ankles, difficulty opening jars, or difficulty carrying an object in their hand. Pain, when present, is usually not well localized and is an aching or cramping feeling.

Myopathies present as *pure motor conditions*, so the classic presentation is weakness without sensory symptoms. On physical examination it is important to assess strength and muscle atrophy. Most myopathies present with *symmetrical proximal weakness*. In some myopathies, ocular and bulbar muscles are affected; this should be noted if present. Sensation should be normal, and reflexes become increasingly diminished as weakness progresses. Contractures of the joints may develop due to loss of strength.

The usual tests ordered to confirm the diagnosis of myopathy include creatine kinase (CK) serum levels (typically elevated), electromyography (EMG), and muscle biopsy. However, it is important to note that other diagnoses, such as motor neuron disease, neuromuscular junction disorders, and sometimes motor neuropathies may mimic myopathies. Therefore, it is usually a good idea to perform nerve conduction studies (NCS) as well as needle study.

Classification

Myopathies can be classified generally as congenital, inflammatory, metabolic, atrophic, or muscular dystrophies (see Table 17.1).

Congenital myopathies. Congenital myopathies typically present in the first few years of life, but occasionally an adult is diagnosed. The clinical symptoms are usually nonspecific. Most of the myopathies in this category have fairly specific histochemical findings when stained, so muscle biopsy is generally needed to confirm the diagnosis.

Inflammatory myopathies. Most inflammatory myopathies are presumably due to some type of immunologic attack of the muscles. However, there are some inflammatory myopathies that are known to be due to infection caused by parasites, viruses, or bacteria.

Metabolic myopathies. These are caused by inherited enzyme deficiencies that are essential for intracellular energy production. Metabolic myopathies may present as typical nonspecific myopathies with proximal weakness as the only clue or with cramps and myoglobinuria. In some cases, metabolic myopathies are part of a more diffuse neurologic syndrome that may involve the central nervous system. Patients may become symptomatic only after exercise. CK levels are typically very elevated.

TABLE 17.1 ■ Examples of Myopathic Disorders

Congenital
Centronuclear myopathy
Myotubular myopathy
Nemaline rod myopathy
Fiber-type disproportion
Inflammatory
Polymyositis
Dermatomyositis
Inclusion body myositis
Viral myopathy (e.g., HIV-associated myopathy/polymyositis and human T-cell lymphotropic virus-I myopathy)
Sarcoid myopathy
Infectious
Trichinosis
Atrophic
Toxic
Colchicine, azidothymidine (AZT), alcohol, chloroquine, hydroxychloroquine, pentazocine, clofibrate, steroids
Endocrine
Thyroid myopathy
Parathyroid myopathy
Adrenal/steroid myopathy
Pituitary myopathy
Metabolic
Acid maltase deficiency myopathy
Carnitine deficiency myopathy
Debrancher deficiency myopathy
Dystrophies
Dystrophin deficiency (Duchenne and Becker)
Facioscapulohumeral muscular dystrophy
Myotonic muscular dystrophy
Emery–Dreifuss muscular dystrophy
Oculopharyngeal muscular dystrophy
Limb girdle muscular dystrophy

Muscular dystrophies. These are inherited muscular disorders, often with an early onset and very progressive course. Some muscular dystrophies can be identified by a specific chromosomal abnormality or gene product (e.g., Duchenne and Becker dystrophy).

Electrodiagnostic Findings

NCS should be *normal.* However, it's usually a good idea to perform a screening. The NCS screen is performed first, and both sensory and motor studies are typically normal. Occasionally in distal myopathies or in severe myopathies that begin proximally but have now affected the distal musculature, the motor NCS may be abnormal. In these cases, the compound muscle action potential (CMAP) amplitudes would be reduced with preserved distal latencies and conduction velocities. A reasonable approach to NCS when assessing for a myopathy would be to perform one motor and one sensory conduction study in both an upper and a lower extremity. EMG plays an important role in the diagnosis of myopathy and is frequently done in conjunction with a muscle biopsy.

EMG not only helps to determine the diagnosis and extent of the disease, but it can also be an important indicator of where the muscle biopsy should be obtained. Needle EMG should not be performed in a muscle that will later be biopsied, as needling may damage the muscle and confuse the biopsy findings.

SENSORY NERVE CONDUCTION STUDIES

Sensory NCSs should be normal in patients with myopathy because sensory fibers are not affected.

MOTOR NERVE CONDUCTION STUDIES

Motor NCSs are typically normal in myopathy, because the active electrode is usually over a *distal* muscle. However, if the myopathy is severe enough to affect both distal and proximal muscles or is one of the less common myopathies that preferentially affect distal muscles, then the motor NCSs may be abnormal. In these cases, there may be evidence of reduced CMAP amplitude. The distal latencies and conduction velocities will be normal because the myelin is not affected.

LATE RESPONSES

Late responses are not usually helpful in myopathies because they are nonspecific.

ELECTROMYOGRAPHY

Myopathies present with characteristic findings on EMG. Myopathic motor units are usually of short duration, small amplitude, and polyphasic and have early recruitment (see Fig. 5.14). This would be seen as a large number of small motor units firing (recruited) during a minimal contraction. The motor unit action potential is typically smaller due to dropout or dysfunction of individual muscle fibers. This leads to a decreased size of the motor unit. The number of motor units usually remains the same except in severe cases where every single fiber drops out and thus eliminates that motor unit.

Spontaneous activity is frequently noted in myopathies. Many myopathies present with positive sharp waves (PSWs) and fibrillation potentials (fibs). Less commonly, myopathies may reveal *myotonic discharges* (see Chapter 5, Electromyography and Chapter 17, Myopathy). It is not uncommon in chronic myopathies to note *complex repetitive discharges*. Rarely there is evidence of *contracture*, which is the *complete absence of electrical activity in the contracted state*.

The EMG study should first focus on the weakest muscles. Typically these are the more proximal muscles. In some instances, the only abnormalities may be in the paraspinal muscles. If these show the typical findings consistent with myopathy, then stronger muscles should be tested as well to determine the extent of the disease. If the clinically weakest muscles are normal, then testing the stronger muscles will not be useful and is not advised. In cases where the muscles show neuropathic instead of myopathic changes, the electromyographer needs to reconsider the scope of the study and expand it to rule out other conditions. In this instance, nerve conduction testing would definitely be indicated. It should also be noted that steroid myopathies predominantly affect Type II fibers. Because EMG testing evaluates Type I fibers, EMG testing is often normal in steroid myopathy.

There are three additional considerations when performing EMG in a suspected myopathic patient. First, it is not a good idea to order a CK blood test shortly after the EMG as the levels may be falsely elevated. Second, when determining which muscle to biopsy, it is wise to choose a muscle that is affected but not completely atrophic. Third, do not test all affected muscles, because once they have been needled, they should not be used for a biopsy. Because EMG can provide important information about which muscles are affected, a good strategy is to biopsy a muscle on the contralateral side of the testing. For example, if the right deltoid is affected on the EMG study, then the biopsy would be on the left deltoid that wasn't tested. The EMG report should clearly identify which muscles have not been tested so that an appropriate decision can be made on which muscle to biopsy.

Summary

In summary, electrodiagnostic findings in myopathy may include:

1. normal SNAP;
2. normal CMAP;
3. spontaneous potentials (PSWs and fibs) in affected muscles; and
4. short-duration, small-amplitude polyphasic motor units with early recruitment in affected muscles on EMG.

CHAPTER 18

Brachial Plexopathies

Julie K. Silver ■ Jay M. Weiss

Clinical Presentation

Evaluation of the brachial plexus is one of the most challenging examinations that the electromyographer will encounter. This is to the result of the complexity of the anatomy and its relative inaccessibility. Moreover, standard nerve conduction protocols do not test many parts of the brachial plexus. A thorough understanding of the anatomy of the brachial plexus is integral to performing an accurate electrodiagnostic study.

Clinical presentations vary according to the area of the brachial plexus that is involved. Most brachial plexus lesions are to the result of trauma. In newborns, obstetrical trauma is the leading cause of injury. In older children or adults, other causes of trauma may involve stretch injuries (e.g., humeral fracture or shoulder dislocation), compression injuries (e.g., seatbelt or backpack straps or a space-occupying lesion such as a tumor), or penetrating injuries (e.g., knife or gunshot wound). The brachial plexus may be affected by space-occupying benign or malignant lesions, or cancer treatment (radiation-induced plexopathy). The majority of brachial plexus lesions in adults are unilateral and affect the dominant limb more commonly than the nondominant limb. Obstetric palsies affect the right side more than the left.

The history and physical examination varies with the type of lesion to the brachial plexus. One useful way to classify the varied brachial plexus lesions is on the basis of their anatomic location. Brachial plexus lesions can be classified into supraclavicular, infraclavicular, and pan plexus lesions (Table 18.1).

The clinical presentation of the lesions of the brachial plexus varies according to the locations involved. For example, injuries to the lateral cord may present with numbness in the lateral aspect of the forearm below the elbow extending just above the thumb. This is the distribution of the *lateral cutaneous nerve of the forearm*. This may be associated with numbness in the distribution of the median nerve (the first, second, and third digits) and with weakness of the biceps, brachioradialis, and pronator teres muscles. A lesion affecting the medial cord may damage the *medial antebrachial cutaneous nerve* and present with numbness of the medial aspect of the forearm. This may be associated with weakness of the flexor carpi ulnaris, abductor pollicis brevis, opponens pollicis, flexor digitorum indicis, abductor digiti minimi, and adductor pollicis muscles.

Brachial plexopathy resulting from metastatic disease in cancer usually presents with severe, intractable pain. Often these lesions are due to spread from an adjacent breast or lung tumor. These plexopathies have a predilection for the lower trunks, but they can also involve a more diffuse pattern. Brachial plexopathy may develop months to years after radiation treatment (e.g., breast, lung, or other cancers that involve chest/mediastinal radiation). Radiation-induced plexopathies are often painful but may be less so than plexopathy due to active cancer. Radiation-induced plexopathies that occur shortly after treatment often have better prognoses than those that develop later. Late onset plexopathies are typically progressive and irreversible. They generally present with paresthesias and sensory loss and tend to be more prominent in the upper trunk distribution. Plexopathies that develop without an obvious antecedent event may be misdiagnosed. For example, because of the lower motor neuron presentation, plexopathies may be mistakenly

TABLE 18.1 ■ Brachial Plexus Lesions

Supraclavicular	Infraclavicular	Pan Plexus
Upper Plexus (Roots/Upper Trunk)	Radiation related	Trauma
Incomplete traction injury	Gunshot wound	Severe traction injury
Erb's palsy	Humeral fracture/dislocation	Late metastatic disease
C5, C6 root avulsions	Dislocation	Late radiation palsy
Axillary nerve block		
Lower Plexus (Roots/Lower Trunk)		
Metastatic tumor		
Pancoast syndrome		
Post sternotomy		
Thoracic outlet syndrome		
Klumpke's palsy (C8, T1)		

diagnosed as amyotrophic lateral sclerosis. Figs. 18.1 and 18.2 review the cutaneous innervation of the extremities.

Anatomy

The brachial plexus (Fig. 18.3) is an intricate neural web that provides the innervation to the upper extremities. Most commonly, the plexus arises from the anterior rami of the C5 to T1 nerves. There are anatomical variants with some patients having contributions from the C4 level or the T2 level. These are known as *prefixed* and *postfixed plexuses*, respectively. The following discussion will focus on the most common pattern of innervation (i.e., C5 to T1).

There are many methods to help learn the anatomy of the plexus. The anatomy need not be intimidating. You can remember the sections of the brachial plexus using the mnemonic, "Robert Taylor Drinks Coors Beer." The mnemonic stands for the five sections of the brachial plexus: roots, trunks, divisions, cords, and branches.

It's often easier to learn the anatomy of the brachial plexus if you sketch it out. To create a schematic of the brachial plexus, start with the five roots, from C5 through T1. Remember that roots C5, C6, and C7 come out above the correspondingly numbered vertebral bodies, C8 exits between C7 and T1 (there is no C8 vertebra), and T1 exits the spine below the T1 vertebra. The *roots* of the plexus originate at the anterior rami of C5 to T1 nerves (Fig. 18.4). The roots run through the anterior and posterior scalene muscles (Fig. 18.5). The C5 and C6 roots join to become the upper trunk. C7 becomes the middle trunk, and C8 and T1 join to become the lower trunk. Connect the roots to the three parallel lines as in Fig. 18.6; these represent the roots and the trunks of the brachial plexus.

The trunks slope down and divide to form the *anterior* and *posterior divisions* (Fig. 18.7). The divisions are found deep under the middle section of the clavicle. They run along a parallel course to the subclavian artery. They then weave around the axillary artery. At this point the posterior divisions of the upper and lower trunks join the middle trunk to form the *posterior cord*. The anterior division of the middle trunk joins the upper trunk fibers to become the lateral cord. At this level the brachial plexus is divided into *lateral, posterior*, and *medial cords* that are named in their relationship to the axillary artery (Fig. 18.8). The brachial plexus then goes on to divide into the terminal nerve branches (Fig. 18.9). The posterior cord becomes the radial nerve but also gives off the axillary nerve. The lateral cord terminates in the *musculocutaneous nerve* and a branch that merges with a branch from the medial cord to form the *median nerve*. So the medial cord terminates by dividing into two main branches: the medial root of the median nerve and the ulnar nerve. The ulnar nerve is composed of fibers that come only from the medial cord, while the other

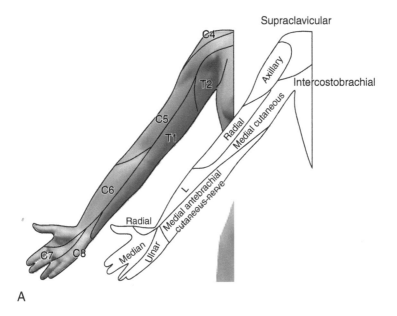

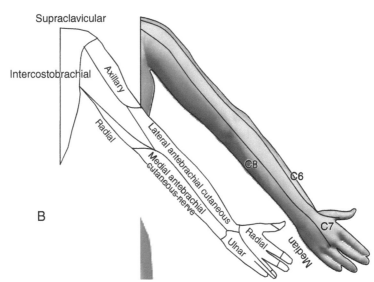

Fig. 18.1 Cutaneous innervation. (A) Volar sensory innervation; (B) dorsal sensory innervation. *L,* Lateral antebrachial cutaneous.

main terminal branch of the medial cord is joined by a branch from the lateral cord to become the median nerve. Because the medial cord does not receive fibers from the upper or middle trunks, all of its fibers originate in the C8 and T1 roots. Because the ulnar nerve is derived solely from the medial cord, all ulnar fibers are from C8 or T1 nerve roots.

In contrast, the median nerve has C8 and T1 fibers (primarily motor to the thenar muscles). It also has motor and sensory fibers from the upper and middle trunks (through the lateral cord) that originated in the C5, C6, and C7 roots, supplying sensation in the hand and primarily forearm flexors.

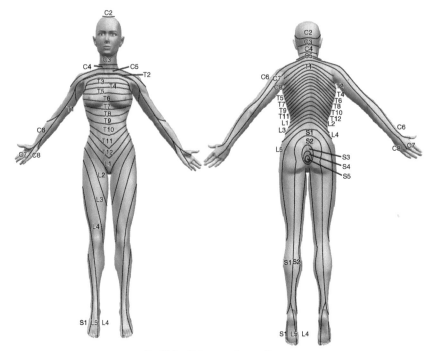

Fig. 18.2 Cutaneous innervation.

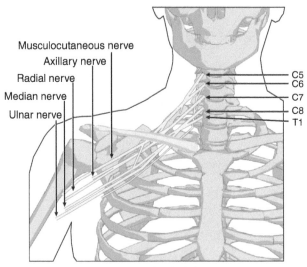

Fig. 18.3 The brachial plexus.

The other main terminal branch in the arm, the radial nerve comes from the posterior cord, which receives fibers from the upper, middle, and lower trunks. Therefore it is composed of fibers from all trunks of the brachial plexus.

Along its course, the brachial plexus gives off *collateral nerves*. These nerves are useful in that they can be used to help localize lesions within or in relation to the brachial plexus. Some of the

Brachial plexus

Roots

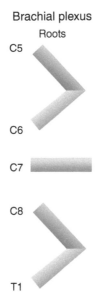

C5

C6

C7

C8

T1

Fig. 18.4   The roots of the brachial plexus.

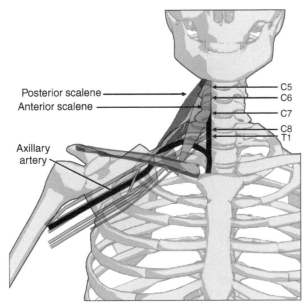

Posterior scalene
Anterior scalene

C5
C6
C7
C8
T1

Axillary
artery

Fig. 18.5   The structure of the brachial plexus.

clinically more important nerves include the *dorsal scapular nerve* to the rhomboids (involvement will localize the lesion above the level of the trunks). The *suprascapular nerve* to the supraspinatus and infraspinatus comes off at the trunk level. For example, plexopathies involving the upper trunk can usually be distinguished from lesions of the lateral cord. Although both will have reduced amplitudes of the musculocutaneous compound muscle action potentials (CMAPs), *lateral antebrachial* sensory nerve action potential (SNAP), and *median* SNAP, only the upper trunk

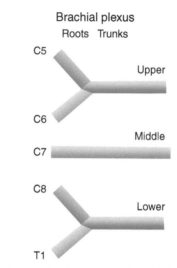

Fig. 18.6   The structure of the brachial plexus.

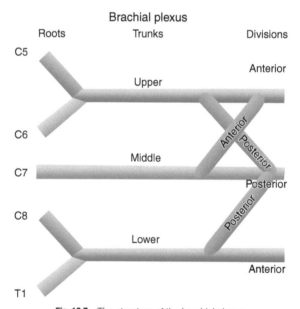

Fig. 18.7   The structure of the brachial plexus.

lesion will have a decreased amplitude of the *axillary nerve* CMAP recorded from the deltoid muscle and *suprascapular* CMAP recorded from the supraspinatus muscle. Only the upper trunk lesion may have spontaneous potentials in the deltoid, brachioradialis, infraspinatus, or supraspinatus muscles. These relationships will be further reviewed in the next section.

TRUNK VERSUS CORD LESIONS

In general, lesions at the trunk and cord levels can appear similar, but there are important differences between the levels. While at first glance a medial cord and a lower trunk lesion or a lateral

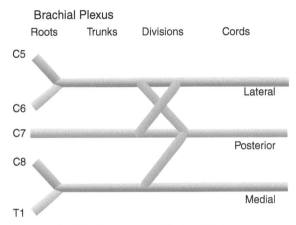

Fig. 18.8   The structure of the brachial plexus.

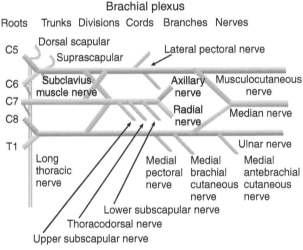

Fig. 18.9   The structure of the brachial plexus.

cord and an upper trunk lesion may appear similar, there are crucial differences in clinical and electromyographic (EMG) appearance that will help with localization.

A lesion at the cord level will generally affect one compartment, such as wrist flexors (in the case of the lateral cord), while at the trunk level, an upper trunk lesion will affect forearm flexors and wrist extensors. Similarly, a posterior cord lesion will affect wrist and finger extensors (and not flexors), while a middle trunk lesion will cause findings in finger and wrist flexors and extensors.

As a general rule, if antagonist muscles are involved, the lesion is at the root or trunk level. If muscles from one compartment are involved without their antagonist muscle, the lesion is at the cord or peripheral nerve level.

Electrodiagnosis

A properly planned and technically correct brachial plexus electrodiagnostic examination can give more information than a physical examination alone. As with all electrodiagnostic studies, this examination should start with a thorough physical examination. A detailed upper extremity neurologic examination will help determine the distribution of motor and sensory abnormalities. When properly planned and clinically guided, the electrodiagnostic examination is the most sensitive physiologic examination of the brachial plexus. This test can help to localize the site of the lesion *and* provide the electromyographer with an estimate of the prognosis of the lesion. When performing an examination to rule out a brachial plexus lesion, it is important to use the unaffected limb as a control and to compare the responses from the two sides.

Examination of the brachial plexus will require learning many nonstandard nerve tests. Standard ulnar and median motor nerve studies examine only nerve fibers from the medial cord and lower trunk. Median sensory nerve studies test fibers from the upper and middle trunks or lateral cord. A brachial plexus lesion is proximal to the segments of these nerves that are being tested. Extensive testing is essential to localize the area of the brachial plexus that is affected and to rule out possible radiculopathies and mononeuropathies as the sources of the patient's symptoms.

Aside from localizing the lesion, the electrodiagnostic test can also establish the severity of nerve damage. Axon loss plexopathy is the most common pattern seen in the electrodiagnostic lab. The electrophysiologic changes depend upon the severity of the axonal loss.

SENSORY NERVE CONDUCTION STUDIES

The sensory nerve conduction study is a more sensitive indicator of injury to the brachial plexus than the motor nerve response. The sensory nerve distal latency and conduction velocity are usually normal in brachial plexus lesions. This is because, in demyelinating lesions, the area of demyelination (causing slowing or conduction block) is proximal to the area being tested. Therefore distal velocities will not be affected. In the case of an axonal lesion, SNAP amplitude may be affected, but velocity and latency will not because the distal nerve and myelin are intact. With mild lesions of the brachial plexus, the SNAP amplitude may be unaffected. With increasing severity of injury to the brachial plexus, the amplitude of the appropriate SNAP may be decreased or absent. The SNAP amplitude reflects the number of functioning axons in continuity with the sensory nerve cell body located in the dorsal root ganglion (Fig. 18.10). Lesions that are proximal to this cell body, such as radiculopathies and nerve root avulsions, do not interfere with the function of the cell body or the sensory nerves derived from that root. Therefore lesions *proximal* to the dorsal root ganglion have intact sensory nerve electrical function, even though sensation may be affected clinically.

Lesions *proximal* to the dorsal root ganglion have a normal SNAP amplitude. Lesions *distal* to the dorsal root ganglion *disconnect the sensory nerve cell body from its axons.* This results in

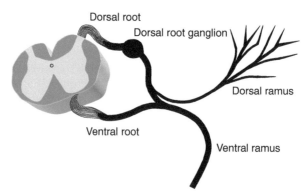

Fig. 18.10 Sensory nerve action potential (SNAP) amplitude may be decreased in lesions affecting the brachial plexus.

deprivation of the axons from their nutritional source. Depending on the severity of the lesion, this may result in a decrement or absence of the SNAP potential. The differentiation between pre- and postganglionic lesions is extremely important. Although both lesions may present with numbness and sensory loss in a defined distribution, the nerve root avulsion (preganglionic lesion) usually portends a poorer prognosis. Such injuries do not undergo spontaneous regeneration and are poorly amenable to surgical repair. The postganglionic lesions have a more favorable prognosis.

MOTOR NERVE CONDUCTION STUDIES

The CMAPs are not affected unless the brachial plexus injury is severe. With severe axonal injuries to the brachial plexus, there may be a reduction in the corresponding CMAP amplitudes. When they are affected, the CMAP is generally a better indication of the extent of axonal loss than SNAP amplitudes.

The motor latencies and conduction velocities are usually unaffected by a brachial plexus lesion because they represent the fibers that are intact (i.e., they do not reflect abnormal conduction across the brachial plexus). However, stimulation across Erb's point (above the lesion) may reveal nerve conduction slowing if there is a demyelinating lesion in the brachial plexus. If a conduction block is present, stimulating across Erb's point may result in a decreased CMAP amplitude (see Chapter 4, Nerve Conduction Studies, for a description of conduction block).

LATE RESPONSES

Most lesions of the brachial plexus are incomplete and have normal conduction across the brachial plexus. The lesion is usually small and localized, so the effect of the slowed segment is diluted along the path of the F-wave. Late responses (F-waves and H-reflexes) are generally not helpful in the evaluation of brachial plexus lesions as they are nonspecific.

ELECTROMYOGRAPHY

Your findings on the history and physical examination will help you decide which muscles to examine with needle EMG. The EMG testing should be mapped out based on a review of the brachial plexus (see Fig. 18.9) before the test is started. Electrodiagnostic findings with acute mild plexopathies are usually limited to fibrillations and positive sharp waves (PSWs) in the muscles innervated by the damaged segment of the plexus. For example, a lesion of the lateral cord may have PSWs noted in the biceps, pronator teres, flexor carpi radialis, and pectoralis muscles. The supraspinatus, infraspinatus, and levator scapulae muscles would be normal. In lesions where reinnervation has occurred, long duration, increased amplitude, or polyphasicity may be noted in the motor unit action potentials.

The clinical manifestations of an injury to the brachial plexus may occur immediately, but the electrodiagnostic findings may take up to 3 weeks to develop. To minimize the likelihood of a false negative study, it is important that the electrodiagnostic test not be performed until 3 weeks after the onset of the injury (if possible), so that sufficient Wallerian degeneration of the distal parts of the injured nerves can occur. This allows for the development of fibrillation potentials (fibs) and PSWs. Testing prior to that time frame may yield confusing and misleading data. Cervical paraspinals are expected to be *normal* in brachial plexus lesions because the paraspinal muscles are innervated by the posterior rami and the brachial plexus is innervated by the anterior rami of the spinal nerve. Table 18.2 maps out important nerve studies and muscles in electrodiagnosis of the brachial plexus. By reviewing the table, you can localize the lesions to the roots or areas of the brachial plexus.

TABLE 18.2 ■ Localization of Lesions in the Brachial Plexus

Anatomical Area of Injury	Affected Sensory NCS	Affected Motor NCS	Positive Findings EMG
Radiculopathy	Normal	CMAPs decreased	Cervical paraspinals Myotomal pattern
Upper trunk	Lateral antebrachial Median nerve to first digit Radial	Musculocutaneous nerve to biceps Suprascapular nerve to supraspinatus Axillary nerve to deltoid	Supraspinatus Biceps Pronator teres Deltoid Brachioradialis
Middle trunk	Median nerve to third and fourth digits	Radial nerve to extensor digitorum communis	Latissimus dorsi Teres major Extensor digitorum communis Pronator teres Flexor carpi radialis
Lower trunk	Ulnar nerve to fifth digit Medial antebrachial	Ulnar nerve to abductor digiti minimi Median nerve to abductor pollicis brevis	Flexor digitorum superficialis Abductor digiti minimi Flexor carpi ulnaris Flexor superficialis Flexor digitorum profundus
Lateral cord	Lateral antebrachial Median nerve to first digit	Musculocutaneous nerve to biceps	Biceps Pronator teres Flexor carpi radialis
Posterior cord	Radial	Axillary nerve to deltoid Radial nerve to extensor carpi ulnaris	Latissimus dorsi Teres major Deltoid Radial muscles
Medial cord	Ulnar nerve to fifth digit Medial antebrachial nerve	Ulnar nerve to abductor digiti minimi Median nerve to abductor pollicis brevis	Ulnar muscles Flexor digitorum superficialis Flexor pollicis longus Abductor pollicis brevis

CMAP, Compound muscle action potential; EMG, electromyography; NCS, nerve conduction study.

Summary

In summary, knowledge of the anatomy of the brachial plexus is crucial in its electrodiagnostic (and clinical) evaluation. Involvement of agonist and antagonist muscles suggests a lesion at the root or trunk level, while involvement limited to one compartment suggests a cord or peripheral nerve lesion.

The electrodiagnostic findings in brachial plexopathy may include (see Table 18.2):
1. decreased SNAP amplitude,
2. decreased CMAP amplitude,
3. slowing of conduction velocity with stimulation across Erb's point,
4. normal EMG findings in the paraspinal muscles, and
5. spontaneous activity (fibs and PSWs) in muscles distal to the level of the injury in muscles innervated by the injured segment.

CHAPTER 19

Lumbosacral Plexopathies

Julie K. Silver ■ Jay M. Weiss

Electrodiagnostic evaluations of the lumbar and sacral plexus (LSP) can be challenging examinations because of the complexity of the anatomy and its relative inaccessibility. Moreover, standard nerve conduction protocols do not test many parts of these areas. A thorough understanding of the anatomy is integral to performing an accurate electrodiagnostic study.

Clinical Presentation

Neurologic damage to the LSP is less common than in the brachial plexus. This is due to the relatively protected position of these neural structures and their decreased vulnerability to injury. Lumbosacral plexopathies can be caused by anatomic injury or abnormalities, such as tumors, hematomas, surgical damage, and trauma. In some cases, it is not the cancer that causes the injury but rather the treatment for the malignancy (radiation plexopathy). In radiation-induced plexopathy, damage to the plexus can occur many years after the cancer treatment. Not surprisingly, in traumatic pelvic fractures, the incidence and severity of injury to the LSP increases with the increasing number of anatomic fractures. The LSP can also be damaged by metabolic insults such as diabetes mellitus, infection, vasculitis, or paraneoplastic syndromes. The presentation of the plexopathy varies according to the structures involved.

Anatomy

The anatomy of the LSPs will be discussed separately. The lumbar plexus (Fig. 19.1) is an intricate neural web that provides innervations to the abdominal wall and the anterior and medial aspect of the thigh. The lumbar plexus is formed in the psoas muscle from the anterior rami of the upper four lumbar nerves L1, L2, L3, and L4. There is sometimes a contribution from T12, but this is variable. The branches of the plexus emerge from the lateral, medial, and anterior borders of the muscle. The iliohypogastric, ilioinguinal, femoral, and lateral femoral cutaneous nerves arise from the lateral aspect of the psoas muscle. The obturator nerve arises from the medial aspect of the psoas muscle. The genitofemoral nerve arises from the anterior aspect of the psoas muscle (Fig. 19.2).

The lumbar plexus has a much simpler pattern than the brachial plexus, because it lacks the distinct subdivisions such as trunks and cords that are characteristic of the brachial plexus. The lumbar plexus consists of anterior primary rami, and these rami divide into anterior and posterior divisions.

Nerve roots from L1, L2, L3, and L4 transverse through the psoas muscle and then coalesce to divide into anterior and posterior divisions. The lumbar plexus then terminates in seven major branches. The first three provide motor and sensory innervation to the abdominal wall and groin. These are the iliohypogastric, ilioinguinal, and genitofemoral nerves. The next three go on to innervate the thigh's anterior and medial aspects. These are the lateral femoral cutaneous, femoral, and obturator nerves. The seventh branch is a contribution from L4 to the sacral plexus. The obturator nerves derive from the anterior divisions. The lateral femoral cutaneous and the femoral

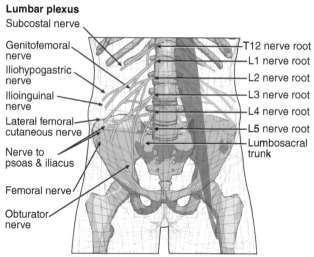

Lumbar plexus

Subcostal nerve

Genitofemoral nerve

Iliohypogastric nerve

Ilioinguinal nerve

Lateral femoral cutaneous nerve

Nerve to psoas & iliacus

Femoral nerve

Obturator nerve

T12 nerve root
L1 nerve root
L2 nerve root
L3 nerve root
L4 nerve root
L5 nerve root
Lumbosacral trunk

Fig. 19.1   Anatomy of the lumbar plexus.

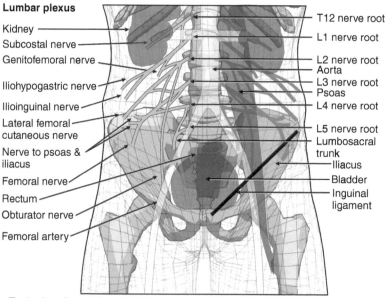

Lumbar plexus

Kidney

Subcostal nerve

Genitofemoral nerve

Iliohypogastric nerve

Ilioinguinal nerve

Lateral femoral cutaneous nerve

Nerve to psoas & iliacus

Femoral nerve

Rectum

Obturator nerve

Femoral artery

T12 nerve root
L1 nerve root
L2 nerve root
Aorta
L3 nerve root
Psoas
L4 nerve root
L5 nerve root
Lumbosacral trunk
Iliacus
Bladder
Inguinal ligament

Fig. 19.2   The lumbar plexus is formed in the psoas muscle from the anterior rami of the upper four lumbar nerves L1, L2, L3, and L4.

nerves arise from the posterior divisions. The femoral nerve terminates in the saphenous nerve, which provides sensation to the medial aspect of the leg. Table 19.1 summarizes the nerves of the lumbar plexus and their respective neural innervation pathways.

The sacral plexus (Figs. 19.3 and 19.4) is similar to the lumbar plexus in that it is primarily a collection of ventral primary spinal nerves that divide into anterior and posterior divisions. These, in turn, divide into multiple peripheral nerves. The sacral plexus provides sensation and muscular and articular innervation to the posterior hip girdle, thigh, and anterior and posterior leg regions.

TABLE 19.1 ■ The Lumbar Plexus

Peripheral Nerve	Root	Division	Sensation	Muscle
Iliohypogastric	L1, L2		Superior gluteal region	None
Genitofemoral	L1, L2		Scrotal skin/adjacent thigh Labia	None
Lateral femoral cutaneous	L2, L3	Posterior	Anterolateral thigh	None
Femoral	L2, L3, L4	Posterior	Anterior thigh Anteromedial thigh Medial leg/foot via the saphenous division of the femoral nerve	Sartorius Iliacus Pectineus Quadriceps
Obturator	L2, L3, L4	Anterior	Medial thigh	Adductor longus Gracilis Adductor brevis Obturator internus Adductor magnus

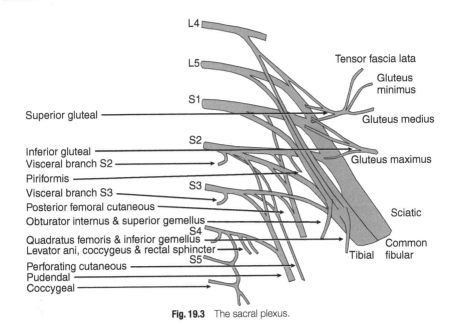

Fig. 19.3   The sacral plexus.

The sacral plexus is composed of primary ventral rami from the L4 to S3 levels. Although the sacral plexus appears intimidating, it is actually quite simple to learn. The plexus is formed in the posterior aspect of the pelvis and lies in the back of the pelvis between the piriformis muscle and the pelvic fascia (see Fig. 19.4).

In front of the sacral plexus are the hypogastric vessels, the ureter, and the sigmoid colon. The superior gluteal and the inferior gluteal vessels run between the first, second, and third sacral nerves, respectively. The close anatomic relationship to these blood vessels makes this structure vulnerable to trauma, which may lead to bleeding and hematoma formation.

The sacral plexus is formed from the ventral primary rami from the L4 through the S3 nerves. All of the nerves (except the S3 root) then divide into an anterior and posterior division.

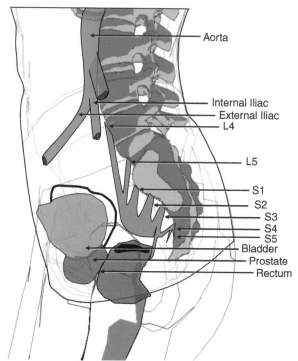

Fig. 19.4 The plexus is formed in the posterior aspect of the pelvis and lies in the back of the pelvis between the piriformis muscle and the pelvic fascia.

The plexus gives off a number of branches, five of which are important to remember for electro-diagnostic testing of this area. The five essential nerves that are critical to keep in mind during the electrodiagnostic evaluation include:

1. superior gluteal nerve,
2. inferior gluteal nerve,
3. posterior femoral cutaneous nerve,
4. sciatic nerve, and
5. pudendal nerve.

The sciatic nerve divides into the fibular and tibial divisions in the thigh. The gluteal, posterior femoral cutaneous, and the common fibular division of the sciatic nerve arise from the posterior components of the sacral plexus. The tibial division of the sciatic nerve, pudendal, and muscular branches to the quadratus femoris, gemellus inferior, obturator internus, and gemellus superior muscles arise from the anterior components of the sacral plexus. Table 19.2 reviews the main contents of the sacral plexus.

Electrodiagnostic Findings

The electrodiagnostic examination is the most sensitive physiologic examination of the lumbosa-cral plexus. This test can help localize the site of the lesion and prognosticate. When performing an examination to rule out a lumbar or sacral lesion, it is important to use the unaffected limb as a control and compare nerve responses from the two sides.

Examination of the lumbosacral plexus may necessitate a few nonstandard nerve tests. For example, the lumbar plexus may require evaluation of the saphenous portion of the femoral nerve,

TABLE 19.2 ■ The Sacral Plexus

Peripheral Nerve	Root	Division	Sensation	Muscle
Superior gluteal	L4, L5, S1	Posterior	None	Gluteus minimus Gluteus medius Tensor fascia lata
Inferior gluteal	L5, S1, S2	Posterior	None	Gluteus maximus
Posterior femoral cutaneous	L2, L3, L4	Posterior	Posterior thigh Scrotum/labia Proximal calf Lower border of gluteus maximus	None
Sciatic (fibular)	L4, L5, S1, S2	Posterior	Posterolateral leg Web space between first and second toes Dorsal/medial leg	Short head of biceps femoris Tibialis anterior Extensor digitorum brevis Peroneus tertius Peroneus brevis Peroneus longus
Sciatic (tibial)	L4, L5, S1, S2, S3	Anterior	Posterior leg Lateral foot Sole of foot	Long head of biceps femoris Semimembranosus Semitendinosus Adductor magnus Plantaris Popliteus Gastrocnemius Tibialis posterior Soleus Flexor digitorum longus Flexor hallucis longus

the lateral femoral cutaneous nerve of the thigh and the femoral nerve. The sacral plexus may require evaluation of the superficial fibular and sural sensory nerves. The fibular motor response from both the extensor digitorum brevis and the tibialis anterior muscles may be required. The tibial response may be recorded from the abductor hallucis and the abductor digiti quinti. Extensive needle electromyography (EMG) is essential to localize the area of the plexus that is affected and to rule out possible radiculopathies or mononeuropathies as the source of the patient's symptoms. Aside from localizing the lesion, the electrodiagnostic test can also establish the severity of nerve damage.

SENSORY NERVE CONDUCTION STUDIES

Sensory nerve studies are more helpful than motor nerve studies in distinguishing plexus lesions from root level lesions. The sensory nerve distal latency and conduction velocity are usually normal in plexus lesions (as the distal segment is normal); however, the sensory nerve action potential (SNAP) amplitude may be decreased in axonal lesions affecting the plexus. With mild lesions of the lumbar or sacral plexus, the SNAP amplitude may be unaffected. With increasing severity of the axonal injury to the plexus, the amplitude of the appropriate SNAPs may be decreased or absent. The SNAP amplitude is a summation of individual functioning sensory axons. For an axon to function, it must be in contact with the sensory nerve cell body. This is located in the dorsal root ganglion (Fig. 19.5).

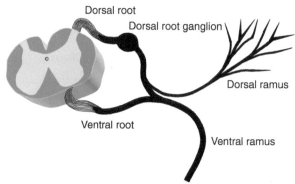

Fig. 19.5   For an axon to function, it must be in contact with the sensory nerve cell body (located in the dorsal root ganglion).

Lesions that are proximal to this cell body, such as radiculopathies and nerve root avulsions, do not interfere with the trophic function of the cell body on the sensory nerves derived from that root. Therefore, lesions proximal to the dorsal root ganglion have intact sensory nerve electrical function. This results in normal SNAP parameters even in the presence of sensory loss. Lesions distal to the dorsal root ganglion disconnect the sensory nerve cell body from its axons. This results in death of the disconnected axons because they are deprived of the nutrition that they need to survive. Depending on the severity of the lesion, this may result in a decrement or absence of the SNAP amplitude. The differentiation of *preganglionic* and *postganglionic* lesions is extremely important. Although both lesions may present with numbness and sensory loss in a defined distribution, the nerve root avulsion usually portends a poorer prognosis because these injuries do not undergo spontaneous regeneration and are usually not amenable to surgical repair. The postganglionic lesions have a more favorable prognosis.

MOTOR NERVE CONDUCTION STUDIES

In general, with lumbosacral plexopathies, the motor latencies and velocities are within normal limits. The compound muscle action potential (CMAP) amplitudes are usually not affected unless the injury is severe. With severe injuries to the plexus, there may be a reduction in the amplitude of the corresponding CMAP. As with the brachial plexus, when CMAP amplitudes are affected, they are generally better indicators of the extent of axonal loss than SNAP abnormalities. Side-to-side amplitude differences can give an approximation of the degree of axonal injury during the first few months following injury. For example, a 70% decrement in CMAP amplitude roughly correlates to a 70% axon loss. The motor latencies and conduction velocities are usually unaffected by a lumbar or sacral lesion because they are a function of the fibers that are intact and do not reflect abnormal conduction across the plexus. One should be cautioned that due to normal aging and day-to-day microtrauma, atrophy of intrinsic foot muscles, and side-to-side amplitude differences are not that unusual with fibular nerve studies, even in asymptomatic individuals. For this reason, amplitude differences of less than 50% may not be significant, depending on the clinical picture.

LATE RESPONSES

Most lesions of the lumbosacral plexus are incomplete and have many areas of normal conduction across the lumbosacral plexus. The lesion may be so localized that the effect of the lesion is not as evident (or *diluted*) along the neural path of transmission of the H-reflex and F-wave. Therefore, H-reflexes and F-waves are usually not helpful in the diagnosis of plexopathies.

ELECTROMYOGRAPHY

Your findings on the history and physical examination will help guide you in determining which muscles to examine electromyographically. Refer to Tables 19.1 and 19.2 to help design your study. Electrodiagnostic findings in plexopathies may include fibrillations (fibs) and positive sharp waves (PSWs) in all muscles innervated distal to the lesion. In chronic lesions, motor unit action potentials (MUAPs) may demonstrate long duration, high amplitude, and polyphasic potentials. Recruitment is usually decreased in all affected muscles.

The clinical manifestations of an injury to the plexus are apparent at onset, but the EMG findings may take up to 3 weeks to develop. It is important that the test be delayed 3 weeks (if possible) after the onset of evidence of nerve involvement so that there will be sufficient time for Wallerian degeneration of the distal parts of the injured nerves to occur; this allows for the development of fibs and PSWs. Testing prior to that time frame can yield confusing and misleading data. Lumbar paraspinals are expected to be normal in LSP lesions because the paraspinal muscles are innervated by the posterior rami, and the plexus is innervated by the anterior rami of the spinal nerve.

A classic lumbar plexus injury may have decreased saphenous, femoral, and lateral femoral cutaneous amplitudes with intact latencies and conduction velocities. In addition, EMG would reveal muscle membrane instability in the vastus medialis obliquus, adductor brevis, sartorius, and iliopsoas. The lumbar paraspinal muscles would test normal in a pure lumbar plexopathy. By using these guidelines, a thorough electrodiagnostic evaluation of the lumbosacral plexus can be planned and carried out with a minimum of discomfort to the patient.

Summary

In summary, the electrodiagnostic findings in lumbosacral plexopathy may include:
1. decreased SNAP amplitude,
2. decreased CMAP amplitude,
3. normal EMG findings in the paraspinal muscles, and
4. abnormal spontaneous activity (fibs and PSWs) in muscles distal to the level of the injury.

CHAPTER 20

Motor Neuron Diseases

Lyn D. Weiss

Motor neuron diseases represent a group of diseases with their primary pathology located in the motor neuron of the brain and/or spinal cord. They therefore can affect both upper and/or lower motor neurons. These disorders include poliomyelitis, amyotrophic lateral sclerosis (ALS), spinal muscular atrophy, primary lateral sclerosis, and progressive bulbar palsy. Although many of these diseases affect both upper and lower motor neurons, only the injury to the lower motor neurons can be assessed with electrodiagnostic testing.

The diagnosis of motor neuron disease is based on the electrodiagnostic findings in conjunction with the physical examination, the neuroimaging, and the laboratory studies. The goal of electrodiagnostic studies is to assess for lower motor neuron dysfunction in clinically affected regions and in regions that are clinically unaffected. The gravity and significance of a diagnosis of motor neuron disease is of such magnitude that if this diagnosis is suspected, referral to a physician with significant experience in this area is recommended.

Clinical Presentation

Patients with motor neuron diseases typically present with findings of both upper and lower motor neuron abnormalities on physical examination. The exceptions to this are poliomyelitis, spinal muscular atrophy, and progressive muscular atrophy, which affect only the lower motor neurons, and primary lateral sclerosis, which affects only the upper motor neurons. Signs and symptoms of upper motor neuron involvement may include spasticity, stiffness, and impaired motor control. Signs and symptoms of lower motor neuron involvement may include muscle atrophy, weakness, flaccidity, fasciculations, and cramps. Four anatomic regions should be assessed clinically and electrodiagnostically: bulbar, cervical, thoracic, and lumbar.

Anatomy

As stated earlier, motor neuron diseases can affect the upper and/or the lower motor neurons. There are usually no significant sensory or cognitive findings.

Electrodiagnostic Findings

SENSORY NERVE CONDUCTION STUDIES

Because motor neuron diseases affect the anterior horn cells and not the dorsal root ganglions, sensory nerve action potentials should show normal amplitude and conduction velocities.

MOTOR NERVE CONDUCTION STUDIES

Compound muscle action potential (CMAP) latencies and conduction velocities should be normal, because the myelin is intact. Because of axonal loss, the amplitude of the CMAPs may be markedly reduced. If there is severe axonal loss, some of the fastest fibers may be lost. Therefore, one may see mildly increased latency and decreased conduction velocity, but the amount of slowing should not exceed about 20% of normal.

LATE RESPONSES

F-waves and H-reflexes are generally not helpful in the diagnosis of motor neuron disease because they are nonspecific.

ELECTROMYOGRAPHY

To diagnose a disease of the anterior horn cells, four anatomic regions should be tested (bulbar, cervical, thoracic, and lumbar). Electrodiagnostic testing often reveals evidence of both acute and chronic changes. Acute findings include spontaneous potentials (fibrillations [fibs] or positive sharp waves [PSWs]) and fasciculation potentials. Chronic neurogenic changes include motor unit action potentials (MUAPs) of long duration, increased polyphasicity, and large amplitude, indicating reinnervation. Decreased recruitment (increased firing frequency of the remaining motor units) should be noted.

Awaji-Shima Criteria

The Awaji-shima criteria help standardize the diagnosis of ALS.[1] This was a consensus recommendation by a panel of experts that modified the El Escorial criteria, which was previously used in the diagnosis of ALS. The Awaji-shima criteria classify the certainty of a diagnosis of ALS into one of three categories: clinically definite, probable, and possible. Clinical evidence of upper and lower motor neuron pathology is sought within each of the four anatomical regions (bulbar, cervical, thoracic, and lumbar). In the Awaji-shima criteria, fasciculation potentials carry the same weight as spontaneous potentials (fibs and PSWs).

Summary

The electrodiagnostic findings in motor neuron diseases may include the following:
1. SNAPs will have normal amplitude and conduction velocity.
2. CMAPs have decreased amplitude with normal (or mildly increased) latency and normal (or mildly decreased) conduction velocity.
3. EMG will demonstrate spontaneous potentials (fibs and PSWs) in affected muscles. Fasciculations and complex repetitive discharges (CRDs) may also be noted. MUAPs may show increased duration, large amplitude, and/or polyphasic potentials if reinnervation has occurred. There will be decreased recruitment as well. Remember to test muscles in all four anatomical regions.

Reference

1. Costa J, Swash M, de Carvalho M. Awaji criteria for the diagnosis of amyotrophic lateral sclerosis: a systemic review. *Arch Neurol*. 2012;69(11):1410–1416.

CHAPTER 21

Critical Illness Neuropathy and Myopathy

Lyn D. Weiss

Introduction

Modern intensive care units (ICUs) have become proficient in increasing the survival of critically ill patients. As medicine advances and more patients survive, an increasing number of them will develop critical illness neuropathy (CIN) and critical illness myopathy (CIM). It should be noted that patients may show evidence of both CIN and CIM.

Critical Illness Neuropathy

CLINICAL PRESENTATION

CIN should be considered in critically ill patients who develop severe weakness, numbness, or difficulty weaning from the ventilator. Often, there is significant muscle atrophy and hyporeflexia.

CIN results in the degeneration of sensory and motor axons. The cause is unknown, although inflammatory cytokines and microvascular dysfunction are believed to be associated with systemic inflammatory response syndrome (SIRS) and lead to axonal degeneration. This degeneration results in an axonal sensory motor neuropathy. Hyperglycemia, hypoalbuminemia, and nutritional factors may increase the risk. Distal fibers are usually affected more than proximal fibers.

Statistically, 47% to 70% of patients admitted to the ICU for sepsis and multiorgan failure have axonal sensorimotor polyneuropathy, which is usually evident within 1 to 3 weeks of admission.[1] Approximately 35% to 50% of these patients have substantial weakness. Extraocular muscles are usually not affected. Cerebrospinal fluid is usually normal or may show mildly elevated protein. CIN is noted mostly in patients with sepsis or SIRS. Hyperglycemia appears to exacerbate the disorder.[2]

ELECTRODIAGNOSTIC MEDICINE EVALUATION

CIN is an axonal sensory motor peripheral neuropathy. The electrodiagnostic evaluation can be quite challenging. Patients often have edema as well as other underlying disorders that may cause neuropathy (e.g., diabetes, thyroid disorders). They may also have cool limbs, which can alter the nerve study results. Factors external to the patient, such as multiple lines, respirators, and increased electrical interference in an ICU setting, can complicate the study. It is important to sample a sufficient number of sensory and motor nerves, and to use multiple stimulation sites in the arms and the legs to get an accurate assessment of whether there is a local or systemic process. This is especially true if edema is present. Nerve conduction testing should *not* be performed if there is an external pacemaker. Sixty cycle electrical interference may be decreased by optimizing electrode (including ground) contacts, by turning on the notch filter, by unplugging the bed, and by turning off unnecessary electrical equipment.

SENSORY NERVE CONDUCTION STUDIES

Sensory nerve conduction studies will show low amplitude or unobtainable sensory nerve action potentials (SNAPs). While there may be mild slowing of the sensory nerve conduction velocities, the decrease in amplitude is usually much more pronounced because this is primarily an axonal process. The slowing may be attributed to loss of the fastest conducting fibers. Distal fibers are usually more affected than proximal fibers.

MOTOR NERVE CONDUCTION STUDIES

Motor nerve conduction studies will show low amplitude or unobtainable compound muscle action potentials (CMAPs). Again, there may be mild slowing of the motor nerve conduction velocities or prolonged distal latencies, but the decrease in amplitude will predominate. The slowing also may be attributed to loss of the fastest conducting fibers. Distal fibers are usually more affected than proximal fibers.

LATE RESPONSES

Late responses (F-waves and H-reflexes) are usually not indicated (and may be technically difficult due to the smaller sizes of these responses). If acute inflammatory demyelinating polyneuropathy (AIDP or Guillain–Barré syndrome) is being ruled out, these studies (particularly F-waves) are important parts of the electrodiagnostic evaluation (see Chapter 22, Inflammatory Neuropathies).

NEEDLE ELECTROMYOGRAPHY

As this type of neuropathy affects the axon, abnormal spontaneous potentials (fibrillations [fibs] and positive sharp waves [PSWs]) may be noted in predominantly distal muscles. Motor units may demonstrate decreased recruitment with increased firing frequency of individual motor units. Chronic changes (nascent reinnervation, or long duration, increased amplitude motor unit action potentials [MUAPs]) may be noted in chronic cases.

CONSIDERATIONS

If a sensory motor axonal peripheral polyneuropathy is noted, the conclusion can stipulate that the test is consistent with CIN. Findings of an axonal sensorimotor neuropathy, however, are not pathognomonic for CIN as it should be noted that other neuropathies (i.e., alcoholic neuropathy) can also present with this pattern of involvement. See Table 16.1 for more information on peripheral neuropathy.

SUMMARY

Patients in the critical care units who have severe weakness, numbness, or difficulty weaning from the ventilator should be considered for CIN.

The classic electrodiagnostic findings in CIN may include:

1. Low amplitude or unobtainable SNAPs
2. Low amplitude or unobtainable CMAPs
3. Needle electromyography (EMG) may show abnormal spontaneous potentials (fibs and PSWs), especially in distal muscles. Motor units may demonstrate decreased recruitment with increased firing frequency of individual motor units. Chronic changes (nascent reinnervation, long duration increased amplitude MUAPs) may be noted in chronic cases.

Critical Illness Myopathy

CLINICAL PRESENTATION

CIM should be considered in critically ill patients who develop severe weakness or difficulty weaning from the ventilator. Patients with CIM usually present with a proximal more than distal flaccid weakness. Because sensory fibers are not involved, sensation should be intact. Reflexes are usually decreased. Facial and extraocular muscles may be affected.

CIM is seen mostly in patients with status asthmaticus, chronic obstructive pulmonary disease (COPD), or liver transplants. There is an association with illness severity, corticosteroid dose, and renal failure. The proposed mechanism for the weakness is reduced excitability of the sarcolemmal membrane.[3]

Approximately 35% of patients with status asthmaticus and COPD will develop CIM.[4] Creatine kinase (CK) levels are usually normal or transiently elevated. Lower corticosteroid dosages may improve the outcome, especially when administrated early in those with refractory shock.[5]

ELECTRODIAGNOSTIC MEDICINE EVALUATION

The electrodiagnostic evaluation should include sensory and motor fibers, as well as a sampling of distal and proximal muscles on needle examination. It is important to note that CIN and CIM can both be present.

SENSORY NERVE CONDUCTION STUDIES

Sensory nerve studies should be normal because sensory fibers are not affected.

MOTOR NERVE CONDUCTION STUDIES

Motor nerve conduction studies are typically normal in patients with CIM. Because myopathies usually affect proximal muscles more than distal muscles, the distal muscles (the ones typically studied on nerve conduction studies) are likely to be normal. In severe cases where significant atrophy is present, the amplitude of the CMAPs may be decreased. Distal latencies and conduction velocities will generally be normal, as the myelin is not affected.

LATE RESPONSES

Late responses (F-waves and H-reflexes) are usually not helpful in the diagnosis of myopathies.

NEEDLE ELECTROMYOGRAPHY

Needle EMG findings are similar to those found in other myopathies. Myopathic motor units typically are of short duration, small amplitude (less than 1 mV), polyphasic, and demonstrate an early recruitment pattern with minimal contraction. Proximal muscles are usually affected more than distal muscles. Spontaneous activity (fibs and PSWs) is frequently noted at rest.

Summary

The classic electrodiagnostic findings in CIM may include:
1. Normal sensory studies (SNAPs).
2. Normal or mildly low amplitude motor studies (CMAPs).
3. Needle EMG may demonstrate spontaneous activity at rest (fibs and PSWs), and MUAPs with short duration, small amplitude, polyphasicity, and early recruitment.

References

1. De Jonghe B, Sharshar T, Lefaucheur JP, et al. Paresis acquired in the intensive care unit: a prospective multicenter study. *JAMA*. 2002;282:2859–2867.
2. Bednarik J, Vondracek P, Dusek L, Moravcova E, Cundrle I. Risk factors for critical illness polyneuromyopathy. *J Neurol*. 2005;252:343–351.
3. Lacomis D. Electrophysiology of neuromuscular disorders in critical illness. *Muscle Nerve*. 2013;47(3): 452–463.
4. Amaya-Villar R, Garnacho-Montero J, Garcia-Garmendia JL, et al. Steroid-induced myopathy in patients intubated due to exacerbation of chronic obstructive pulmonary disease. *Intensive Care Med*. 2005;31: 157–161.
5. Kox M, Pickkers P. "Less is more" in critically ill patients: not too intensive. *JAMA Intern Med*. 2013;173: 1369–1372.

CHAPTER *22*

Inflammatory Neuropathies

Lyn D. Weiss

Inflammatory neuropathies represent a spectrum of peripheral neuropathies that result from an inflammatory response. They are frequently categorized based on whether the symptoms are acute or chronic. Guillain–Barré syndrome (GBS), also known as acute inflammatory demyelinating polyneuropathy (AIDP), and its variants are the most common of the inflammatory neuropathies. Chronic inflammatory neuropathies include chronic inflammatory demyelinating polyneuropathy (CIDP) and multifocal motor neuropathy (MMN). Although the immune reaction is usually directed against the myelin producing Schwann cells, the axons can be affected as well.

Clinical Presentation

The clinical presentation depends upon whether the inflammatory neuropathy is acute or chronic. In AIDP, patients typically develop an acute progressive symmetric weakness. Facial, respiratory and bulbar muscles may be affected. The symptoms usually begin in the legs. Reflexes are generally absent. Respiratory function can be compromised, and 10% to 30% of patients may require ventilatory support. Autonomic dysfunction may also be present and can include tachycardia, urinary retention, hypertension, hypotension, orthostatic hypotension, bradycardia, arrhythmias, and ileus. For these reasons, patients are often admitted and monitored in an intensive care unit setting. Sensory symptoms are usually mild, and pain occurs in about 66% of patients. The symptoms progress over about 2 weeks. Approximately 90% of patients reach their nadir by 4 weeks after the onset of symptoms.

CIDP can initially present identically to AIDP. In the first 2 months, it may be difficult to distinguish CIDP from AIDP. If the disease progresses for more than 8 weeks or if the patient relapses, CIDP should be considered. The differentiation of AIDP and CIDP is made based primarily on the temporal presentation. This can be an important distinction because, even though these are both inflammatory neuropathies, different treatment approaches may be recommended.

There are several variants of AIDP, including Miller Fisher syndrome (ophthalmoplegia, ataxia, and areflexia), as well as axonal forms.

MMN is a chronic inflammatory neuropathy that presents as purely a motor disorder with asymmetric weakness. This neuropathy will involve some motor nerves and spare others. Sensory nerves are not affected, and patients typically do not have sensory abnormalities. The presentation of pure motor weakness may suggest amyotrophic lateral sclerosis, but there are no upper motor neuron findings such as hyperreflexia.

Pathogenesis

Patients will frequently have an antecedent infection. The predominant theory is that the infection evokes an immune response, which in turn cross-reacts with peripheral nerve components due to sharing of cross-reactive epitopes. Two-thirds of patients report antecedent respiratory or gastrointestinal infections (especially *Campylobacter jejuni*). Whereas a link was once noted between vaccines and AIDP, a recent 12-year retrospective study found no link between AIDP and flu vaccine or other vaccines.[1] It is hypothesized that previous vaccine links to GBS may have been due to previously used production techniques.

Anatomy and Laboratory Findings

Patients with AIDP will have elevated cerebral spinal fluid protein with normal white blood cell count. Glycolipid antibodies may be noted. In AIDP, the immune reaction is directed against epitopes in Schwann cell surface membranes or myelin. In the axonal form of AIDP, the immune reaction is directed against epitopes in the axonal membrane. In Miller Fisher syndrome, the immune reaction is directed against GQ1v (ganglioside component of the nerve). In MMN, anti–GM 1 antibodies are present in 50% to 60% of patients.[2] Axonal findings portend a poorer prognosis.

Electrodiagnostic Findings

The electrodiagnostic findings will depend on which structure (axon, myelin) is more affected by the autoimmune process. It will also depend on the segment of the nerve involved. The root is frequently involved, and some may refer to this as a polyradiculoneuropathy as it can have primarily proximal involvement.

SENSORY NERVE CONDUCTION STUDIES

Absent or slowed conduction velocities may be noted in the sensory nerve action potentials. Sural nerves may be spared. (In MMN, sensory studies are normal.)

MOTOR NERVE CONDUCTION STUDIES

Motor nerve conduction studies usually show increased distal latencies, conduction block, nerve conduction velocity slowing, and temporal dispersion (see Chapter 4, Nerve Conduction Studies). These findings reflect the multifocal, widespread patchy distribution of findings. Facial nerve conduction studies and blink reflexes may be helpful.

LATE RESPONSES

One of the rare indications for performing F-waves is suspected AIDP. As the lesions can affect parts of the nerve and miss other segments, F-waves (by virtue of their ability to test the entire length of the nerve) are particularly useful, while short segment studies may be completely normal. Furthermore the inflammatory process frequently begins at the nerve roots, which cannot be assessed by more conventional nerve study techniques. Absent or prolonged F-waves are usually the earliest findings. F-ratios may show an increased ratio, indicating a slowing of the proximal compared to the distal segment (see Chapter 4, Nerve Conduction Studies).

NEEDLE ELECTROMYOGRAPHY

In most cases of AIDP and CIDP there is demyelination, but minimal or no axonal injury. This typically would present on needle EMG as decreased recruitment, without significant abnormal spontaneous potentials. If axonal damage is present, patients may present with findings suggesting denervation on needle EMG testing (provided the test is performed within the appropriate time frame of about 3 weeks from the onset of symptoms).

Summary

1. The earliest findings in AIDP are prolonged or absent F-waves.
2. Prolonged distal latencies, conduction block, conduction velocity slowing, and temporal dispersion may be noted with demyelinating AIDP.
3. Axonal degeneration may be present; needle testing may show denervation.
4. Serial EMGs may be helpful to prognosticate, follow the disease progression, and/or diagnose any associated neurologic conditions.

References

1. Baxter R, Bakshi N, Fireman B, et al. Lack of association of Guillain–Barré syndrome with vaccinations. *Clin Infect Dis.* 2013;57(2):197–204.
2. Vernino S. Antibody testing in peripheral neuropathies. *Neurol Clin.* 2007;25(1):29–46.

CHAPTER 23

Neuromuscular Junction Disorders

Lyn D. Weiss

Introduction

The neuromuscular junction (NMJ) is the relay between the nerve terminal and the skeletal muscle fiber. Chemical transmission across the synaptic cleft is via acetylcholine (ACh). Disorders of the NMJ can be classified into immune mediated, metabolic, toxic, or congenital. The three most common NMJ disorders are myasthenia gravis (MG), Lambert–Eaton myasthenic syndrome (LEMS), and botulism. Disorders can further be classified as affecting the postsynaptic membrane (MG) or the presynaptic membrane (LEMS and botulism). See Table 23.1.

Clinical Presentation

NMJ disorders spare the sensory nerves because only the NMJ is affected. Therefore, sensation is usually intact. Proximal muscles are usually affected more than distal muscles, and bulbar or extraocular muscles may be affected as well. Patients with MG may complain of muscle fatigue that improves with rest. Associated disorders include a 15% incidence of thymoma in patients with MG and a 60% and 70% association of paraneoplastic syndrome (small-cell carcinoma) in patients with LEMS. Botulism is caused by the toxin produced by the bacteria *Clostridium botulinum*. As this is a very rare disorder, a detailed discussion of botulism is beyond the scope of this text. However, as this toxin blocks the presynaptic release of ACh, its electrodiagnostic presentation is similar to LEMS. Most cases of botulism in the US are infantile botulism, with the GI tract colonized by the *Clostridium* bacteria. Wound infection with *Clostridium* bacteria causing botulism is less common.

Electrodiagnostic Medicine Evaluation

In a patient with a suspected NMJ disorder, repetitive nerve stimulation (RNS) and exercise testing should be performed in addition to routine nerve conduction studies (NCSs) and electromyography (EMG). Single-fiber EMG testing can be performed, but a discussion of how to perform this test is beyond the scope of this text. Anticholinesterase medication should be withdrawn 8 to 24 hours prior to testing.

SENSORY NERVE CONDUCTION STUDIES

Because only the NMJ is affected, sensory studies should be normal. It is important to perform sensory studies to confirm that they are indeed normal.

MOTOR NERVE CONDUCTION STUDIES

Motor NCSs will usually have normal latencies and conduction velocities, as the myelin is not affected in disorders of the NMJ. In MG, motor nerve amplitudes are usually preserved. In LEMS, baseline compound muscle action potential (CMAP) amplitudes are usually very low (about 10% of normal).

TABLE 23.1 ■ Comparison of Myasthenia Gravis (MG) and Lambert–Eaton Myasthenic Syndrome (LEMS)

	MG	LEMS
Clinical		
Limb weakness	Proximally predominant	Proximal but more diffuse
Bulbar weakness	Common	Less common
Repetitive contraction	Fatigable	Potentiates strength
Sensory	Normal	May be involved
Reflexes	Normal	Reduced, potentiated with exercise
Dysautonomia	Absent	Present
Pathophysiology		
Site	Postsynaptic	Presynaptic
Antibody	Acetylcholine receptor	Voltage-gated calcium channel
Repetitive Nerve Stimulation		
Baseline compound muscle action potential (CMAP)	Normal	Reduced
Decrement at rest	None at rest if mild	Usually
Brief exercise (10 seconds)	Repair if decrement at rest	Facilitation
1 minute exercise	Repair if decrement at rest	May miss facilitation
2–5 minutes postexercise	Postexercise exhaustion	Postexercise exhaustion
Needle electromyography (EMG)		
Fibrillation potentials	Rare unless severe	Rare unless severe
Motor unit action potentials (MUAPs)	Varying (more at higher rates) Occasionally myopathic	Varying (less at higher rates) Occasionally myopathic

REPETITIVE NERVE STIMULATION

RNS should be performed in both a proximal motor nerve and a distal motor nerve. It is technically easier to study distal muscles, but proximal muscles are more likely to have an abnormal result. It is important that the limb be immobilized and the temperature maintained (32°C in the upper extremities and 30°C in the lower extremities).

RNS is performed using supramaximal stimulation. The nerve is stimulated five times at a rate of 3 Hz. In normal muscles, there is little or no decrement from the first to the fifth stimulation. A decrement of more than 10% from the first to the fifth stimulations is considered significant and may indicate MG (Fig. 23.1).

EXERCISE TESTING

In patients with suspected NMJ disorders, it is important to repeat the repetitive nerve stimulation immediately after 10 seconds of maximal muscle contraction (looking for postactivation facilitation) and then every minute for 3 to 4 minutes (looking for postactivation exhaustion). This exercise may be performed by maximally contracting the muscle or by stimulating the muscle at 50 Hz. In LEMS, although baseline CMAP amplitudes are very low, there is a significant postactivation potentiation (calcium influx facilitates transmitter release). CMAP amplitudes may increase by more than 200% when RNS is performed immediately after exercise. In MG, even if the RNS at rest does not show changes, there may be a CMAP decrement due to postexercise exhaustion.

LATE RESPONSES

Late responses (F-waves and H-reflexes) are not indicated, as they do not provide any additional information.

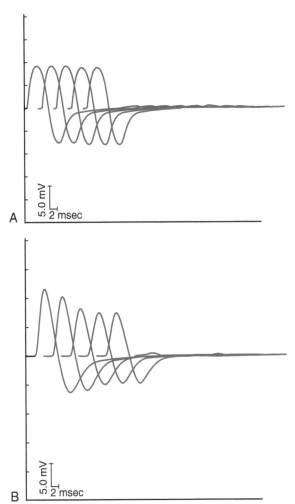

Fig. 23.1   (A) Normal repetitive nerve stimulation (RNS); (B) decrement in amplitude noted from the first to the fifth stimulations.

NEEDLE ELECTROMYOGRAPHY

Weak muscles should be included in EMG testing. Motor unit action potentials (MUAPs) may show abnormalities such as instability (MUAPs that change in configuration). A trigger and delay line may be needed to track the stability of individual motor units (see Chapter 3, About the Machine). This is the result of the blocking of individual muscle fibers. Loss of individual myofibers may result in short-duration, low-amplitude MUAPs, which can be confused with a myopathic process. Abnormal spontaneous activity is usually not noted in NMJ disorders, with the exception of botulism.

Summary

In summary, electrodiagnostic findings in NMJ disorders may include:
1. Sensory nerve action potentials should be normal. (Sensory fibers are not affected as this disorder affects the NMJ.)

2. Motor studies should demonstrate normal latency and conduction velocity as myelin is normal. CMAP amplitudes are usually normal, except in LEMS, where baseline amplitudes are very low.
3. More than 10% decrement in amplitude of CMAP with RNS.
4. Postactivation facilitation may be noted in patients with LEMS (large increase in CMAP amplitude after maximal muscle contraction). In patients with suspected MG and normal RNS, repeat the RNS after exercise and then at 1-minute intervals to assess for decrement in amplitude (postexercise exhaustion).
5. Needle EMG of distal and proximal muscles may display unstable MUAPs with normal recruitment.

CHAPTER 24

How to Write a Report

Lyn D. Weiss

Documentation is a critical part of performing electrodiagnostic studies. Writing a meaningful report will convey your findings to the referring physician and will help determine future testing or treatments. Reports may be used in deciding work-related claims or may become an official part of legal proceedings. Proper documentation is also an essential part of third-party payer reimbursement for electrodiagnostic studies. Most reports contain the following information:

1. Patient's name, identification number (if applicable), date of test, name of physician performing the test, and referring physician.
2. Brief history (including reason for referral or clinical question being asked) and physical examination (including, at a minimum, a focused neurologic assessment).
3. Table of results, including nerve tracings. This is important in case the test needs to be repeated at a later date. Results can be compared for electrophysiologic improvement or progression.
4. Results: the pertinent findings should be discussed. Specific nerve or muscle abnormalities can be discussed.
5. Conclusion: the conclusion should address the reason for the referral (is the suspected diagnosis confirmed?) and the final electrophysiologic diagnosis.

Findings

For each motor nerve tested, the latency, amplitude (and/or area under the curve), and conduction velocity should be reported. Since the tabular data is usually included as part of the report, specific numbers are usually not necessary in this section of the report. It is helpful if the tabular printout flags abnormal values or labels individual nerve latencies, velocities, or amplitudes as increased, decreased, or normal. Abnormal findings should be highlighted in this area. Abnormalities can be recorded as increased or decreased. In instances of severe abnormalities, when a number is far outside the normal range (i.e., a median distal motor latency of 8.2 msec or an amplitude decrement of 80%), it would be appropriate to mention it in the findings section.

For each sensory nerve tested, amplitude and distal latency or conduction velocity should be recorded. Once again, if this is a tabular printout, these do not need to be listed. Abnormalities, however, should be noted. These can be reported as increased or decreased. Since we are usually determining the sensory conduction velocity based on the latency, it is imperative to accurately measure the distance from the stimulator to the recording electrode. It should be noted whether the latency was measured to peak or onset.

ELECTROMYOGRAPHIC FINDINGS

For electromyographic findings, report on insertional activity, activity at rest, motor unit action potential (MUAP) morphology and recruitment.

Insertional Activity

Insertional activity is due to the mechanical depolarization of muscle fibers due to needle insertion and movement. It is normal to have some insertional activity. However, the activity should cease almost immediately following cessation of needle movement. Increased insertional activity exists when there is a run of fibrillation potentials (fibs) or positive sharp waves (PSWs) that only briefly persist beyond needle movement. (To be considered true fibs or PSWs, the waves should persist beyond 0.5 to 1 second.) This is a somewhat subjective component, and its accurate determination is dependent on the experience of the electromyographer. Myotonic discharges or other abnormal potentials may also be noted on insertional activity.

Spontaneous Activity

There is a variety of potentials that may be noted when the needle is at rest in the muscle. These potentials (and their significance) are described in Chapter 5, Electromyography (Table 24.1).

Motor Unit Action Potentials

MUAPs should be classified as normal or abnormal based on their morphology (appearance). If abnormal, the reason for the abnormality should be indicated. Abnormalities could include duration, phases, and/or amplitude.

Motor Unit Recruitment

Recruitment abnormalities should be noted. For example, if there are few functioning motor units the remaining functioning units will fire at a higher frequency without other units being recruited. This abnormal (decreased recruitment or increased firing frequency) should be noted.

Table 24.2 summarizes the findings to be reported on a nerve conduction studies/electromyography report.

Conclusion

Once you have completed a thorough electrodiagnostic examination, you want the pertinent information relayed to the referring physician. The conclusion should summarize your findings. Pertinent negative findings are also important. For example, a referring physician is requesting an electromyogram to rule out carpal tunnel syndrome. You find no evidence of carpal tunnel syndrome, but you do find a C6 radiculopathy. It would be important to note that there is no electrodiagnostic evidence of carpal tunnel syndrome (a negative finding), and there is

---

TABLE 24.1 ■ **Types of Spontaneous Activity**

- Regular Firing
  - Fibrillation potentials (fibs) and positive sharp waves (PSWs)
  - Complex repetitive discharges (CRDs)
  - Myotonic (wax and wane)
- Irregular (random Change)
  - Endplate spikes
  - Fasciculation potentials
- Semi-Rhythmic
  - Motor units (voluntary control)
- Bursts
  - Myokymic discharges
  - Spasm and tremor

TABLE 24.2 ■ Electromyography/Nerve Conduction Study Reporting

Motor Nerves
A. Latency
B. Amplitude
C. Conduction velocity

Sensory Nerves
A. Amplitude
B. Conduction velocity or distal latency

Needle Study
A. Insertional activity
　Increased (denervated muscle, myotonic discharges)
　Decreased (atrophy)
　Normal
B. Spontaneous activity
　Fibrillation potentials (fibs)
　Positive sharp waves (PSWs)
　Myotonic discharges
　Complex repetitive discharges (CRDs)
　Fasciculations
　Myokymic discharges
　Cramps
　Neuromyotonic discharges
　Tremor
　Multiples
C. Motor unit action potential (MUAP) morphology
　Duration
　Polyphasicity
　Amplitude
D. Recruitment
　Increased firing frequency (decreased recruitment)
　Early
　Normal

SAMPLE REPORT

UNIVERSITY MEDICAL CENTER
Department of Physical Medicine and Rehabilitation
Anytown, N.Y.
(516) 123-4567

Patient: Mary Smith　　**DOB:** 2/1/54　　**Physician:** A. Attending
MR#: 1234567　　**Sex:** Female　　**Resident:** A. Resident
Ref Phys: Dr. Jones　　**Test date:** ••/••/20••

Patient History:
This is an ••-year-old female with a chief complaint of a morning pain in her right hand and tingling sensation in the right 1–3 digits for the last 2–3 months. Past medical history was significant for a whiplash injury about 3 years ago. She was seen at this hospital after the motor vehicle accident and discharged home on the same day. She doesn't take any medications except over-the-counter 'pain killers' and Lipitor for cholesterol control. The patient is right-handed. She works as a housekeeper. NCS/EMG was requested by her primary care physician to rule out right carpal tunnel syndrome.

Physical Examination:
Upon physical examination, the patient appeared alert and oriented to person, place, and time and was in no acute distress. There was no atrophy noted in bilateral thenar and hypothenar regions. There was full range of motion of both upper extremities. Motor exam of bilateral upper extremities revealed 5/5 strength in all upper extremity muscles, except right grip was 4/5. There was a positive Tinel's sign elicited at the right wrist. Phalen's test was positive on the right. Upon cervical examination there was very mild paravertebral muscle spasm bilaterally. Spurling's test was negative bilaterally.

Fig. 24.1 Sample report.

SAMPLE REPORT (Continued)

ELECTRODIAGNOSTIC RESULTS

Site	NR	Onset (ms)	Norm Onset (ms)	O–P Amp (mV)	Norm Amp (mV)	Segment Name	Dist (cm)	Vel (m/s)	Norm Vel (m/s)
Left Median (Abd Poll Brev)									
Wrist		3.36	<4.2	10.43	>4.0	Elbow–Wrist	18.5	52.56	>50.0
Elbow		6.88		11.00	>4.0				
Right Median (Abd Poll Brev)									
Wrist		4.61	<4.2	12.00	>4.0	Elbow–Wrist	16	46.51	>50.0
Elbow		8.05		12.34	>4.0				
Left Ulnar (Abd Dig Min)									
Wrist		2.81	<3.4	9.19	>4.0	B Elbow–Wrist	15	64.10	>50.0
B Elbow		5.16		6.02	>4.0	A Elbow–B Elbow	12	85.11	>50.0
A Elbow		6.56		9.89	>4.0				
Right Ulnar (Abd Dig Min)									
Wrist		3.13	<3.4	8.68	>4.0	B Elbow–Wrist	15.5	62.00	>50.0
B Elbow		5.63		10.11	>4.0	A Elbow–B Elbow	12	66.67	>50.0
A Elbow		7.42		9.80	>4.0				

SAMPLE REPORT

				Sensory Nerves					
Site	NR	Onset (ms)	Norm Onset (ms)	O–P Amp (μV)	Norm Amp (μV)	Segment Name	Dist (cm)	Vel (m/s)	Norm Vel (m/s)
Left Median Sen D2 (2nd Digit)									
Mid Palm		0.91		50.21	>20.0	Mid Palm–2nd Digit	6	65.93	>45.0
Wrist		2.28		38.20	>20.0	Wrist–2nd Digit	12	52.63	>44.0
Right Median Sen D2 (2nd Digit)									
Mid Palm		0.88		43.01	>20.0	Mid Palm–2nd Digit	6	68.18	>45.0
Wrist		3.09		18.34	>20.0	Wrist–2nd Digit	12	38.83	>44.0
Left Ulnar Sen (5th Digit)									
Wrist		2.34		23.53	>18.0	Wrist–5th Digit	14.0	59.83	
Right Ulnar Sen (5th Digit)									
Wrist		2.47		24.52	>18.0	Wrist–5th Digit	14.0	56.68	

				EMG							
Side	Muscle	Nerve	Root	Ins Act	PSW	Fibs	Amp	Poly	Fascic	Recrt	Pt Coop	Comment
Right	Abd Poll Brev	Median	C8–T1	Nml	0	0	Nml	0	0	Nml	Nml	
Right	1st Dor Int	Ulnar	C8–T1	Nml	0	0	Nml	0	0	Nml	Nml	
Right	Cerv Para C6	Rami	C6	Nml	0	0	Nml	0	0	Nml	Nml	
Right	Cerv Para C7	Rami	C7	Nml	0	0	Nml	0	0	Nml	Nml	

Electrodiagnostic Evaluation:
Nerve conduction study of the motor and sensory divisions of bilateral median and ulnar nerves was done. Right median compound muscle action potential (CMAP) showed increased distal latency with normal amplitude and conduction velocity. The left median and bilateral ulnar nerve CMAPs showed normal distal latency, amplitude, and conduction velocity.

Right median sensory nerve action potential (SNAP) showed decreased amplitude and slowed conduction velocity across the wrist. The left median and bilateral ulnar SNAPs showed normal amplitude and conduction velocity.

Monopolar needle EMG of the right cervical paraspinal muscles and right abductor pollicis brevis and first dorsal interosseous muscles was performed. EMG of the muscles showed normal insertional activity with no spontaneous activity at rest, normal motor unit action potential morphology and normal recruitment pattern.

Impression:
This study showed electrodiagnostic evidence of right median nerve demyelinating neuropathy across the carpal tunnel involving both motor and sensory fibers. There is no electrodiagnostic evidence of denervation in the right abductor pollicis brevis muscle. This is consistent with mild-to-moderate right carpal tunnel syndrome.

Thank you for the courtesy of this referral.

A. Resident, MD
Resident Physician

I have performed this test with the resident and agree with the above interpretation and conclusion.

A. Attending, MD
Attending Physician

Fig. 24.1 (Continued)

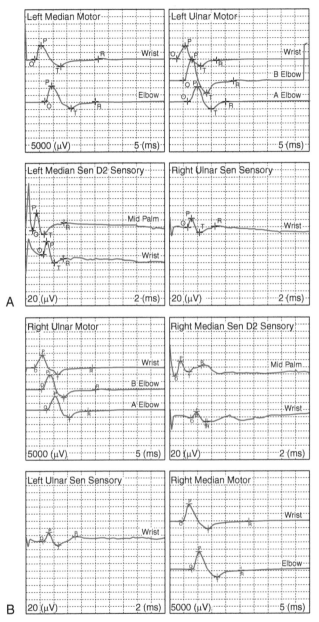

Fig. 24.1 (Continued)

electrodiagnostic evidence of a C6 cervical radiculopathy (a positive finding). (The term *electrodiagnostic evidence* is important because, although there may be clinical signs of a disorder, your conclusion should only report what the electrodiagnostic test reveals.)

Suggestions for possible treatments or interventions can be included in the report, but it is up to the referring physician to implement those suggestions. If further electrodiagnostic testing is indicated at a later time to help prognosticate, this should also be documented in the conclusion.

The sample report (Fig. 24.1) is an example of how electrodiagnostic reports can be written.

CHAPTER 25

Tables of Normals

Lyn D. Weiss

It should be noted that each electrodiagnostic laboratory should develop its own standardized normal values. These tables should be used as references.

TABLE 25.1 ■ Upper Extremity—Motor

Nerve	Recording Electrode	Stimulation Site	Distance (cm) From Active to First Stimulation Site	Onset Latency (msec)	Amplitude (mV)[a]	Segment Name	Velocity (m/sec)
Median	Abductor pollicis brevis	Wrist	8	<4.2	>4.0	Elbow–wrist	>50
		Elbow	TBD[b]		>4.0		
Ulnar	Abductor digiti minimi	Wrist	8	<3.4	>4.0		
		Below elbow (BE)	TBD[b]		>4.0	BE–wrist	>50
		Above elbow (AE)	TBD[b]		>4.0	AE–BE	>50
Radial	Extensor indicis proprius (EIP)	Forearm	4	<2.9	>3.0	AE–EIP	>50
		Erb's point	TBD[b]			Erb's point–AE	>55

[a]Side-to-side amplitude difference of > 50% is significant, or > 20% amplitude drop distal to proximal is significant.
[b]TBD = distance to be determined by the surface measurement.
Skin temperature should be maintained at 32°C. Distances may need to be modified based on size.

TABLE 25.2 ■ Upper Extremity—Sensory

Nerve	Recording Electrode	Stimulation Site	Distance (cm)	Onset Latency (msec)	Amplitude (µV)	Segment Name	Velocity (m/sec)
Median	Second digit	Mid palm	7	<1.9	>20	Mid palm–second digit	>45
		Wrist	14 (7 from palm)	<3.5	>20	Wrist–mid palm	>45
Ulnar	Fifth digit	Wrist	14	<3.1	>18	Wrist–fifth digit	>44
Radial	First digit	wrist	10		>10		

Skin temperature should be maintained at 32°C.

TABLE 25.3 ■ Lower Extremity—Motor

Nerve	Recording Electrode	Stimulation Site	Distance (cm)	Onset Latency (msec)	Amplitude (mV)	Segment Name	Velocity (m/sec)
Fibular	Extensor digitorum brevis	Ankle Fibular head	8	<5.5	>2.5	Fibular head–ankle	>40
		Popliteal				Popliteal–fibular head	>40
Tibial							
Medial plantar	Abductor hallucis	Ankle Knee	10	<6.0	>3.0	Knee–ankle	>40
Lateral plantar	Abductor digiti minimi	Ankle	10	<6.0	>3.0		

Skin temperature should be maintained at 30°C. As in the hand, distances may need to be modified based on size.

TABLE 25.4 ■ Lower Extremity—Sensory

Nerve	Recording Electrode	Stimulation Site	Distance (cm)	Onset Latency (msec)	Amplitude (µV)	Segment Name	Velocity (m/sec)
Sural	Lateral malleolus	Calf	14	<3.8	>10.0	Calf–lateral malleolus	>36
Lateral femoral cutaneous	1 cm medial to the anterior superior iliac spine (ASIS)	Anterior thigh	12–16	2.6 ± 0.2	10–25	ASIS–anterior thigh	>44
Superficial fibular	Anterior to lateral malleolus	Anterolateral calf	14	3.4 ± 0.4	18.3 ± 8.0	Lateral malleolus to calf	51.2±5.7

Skin temperature should be maintained at 30°C.

TABLE 25.5 ■ H-Reflex (See Table 4.1—Nomogram for Normal Values)

Site	Recording Electrode	Latency (msec)	Stimulation Site
Medial gastrocnemius soleus muscle	Halfway from mid popliteal crease—proximal flare medial malleolus	28.0–35.0	Popliteal fossa (cathode proximal) use submaximal stimulation

Skin temperature should be maintained at 30°C.

TABLE 25.6 ■ F-Waves and F-Ratio—Upper Extremities

Motor Nerve	Recording Electrode	F-Latency (msec)	F-Ratio[a]
Median	Abductor pollicis brevis	Wrist 29.1 ± 2.3 Elbow 24.8 ± 2.0 Axilla 21.7 ± 2.8	0.7<F<1.3
Ulnar	Abductor digiti minimi	Wrist 30.5 ± 3.0 BE 26.0 ± 2.0 AE 23.5 ± 2.0 Axilla 11.2 ± 1.0	0.7<F<1.3
Fibular	Extensor digitorum brevis	Ankle 51.3 ± 4.7 Knee 42.7 ± 4.0	0.7<F<1.3
Tibial	Abductor hallucis	Ankle 52.3 ± 4.3 Knee 43.5 ± 3.4	0.7<F<1.3

[a]F-ratio $= \dfrac{F - M - 1}{2M}$ (as measured with elbow or knee stimulation)
where F = F-wave latency and M = wave latency.
AE, Above elbow; *BE*, below elbow.

TABLE 25.7 ■ Significant Differences (Side-to-Side or Nerve-to-Nerve)

Median-to-ulnar distal motor latency	>1 msec	Consider carpal tunnel syndrome.
Median-to-ulnar distal sensory latency	>0.5 msec	Consider carpal tunnel syndrome.
Combined sensory index (CSI)[a]	>0.9 msec	Consider carpal tunnel syndrome.
H-reflex side-to-side difference	>1.5 msec	Consider S1 radiculopathy.
Proximal-to-distal drop in motor amplitude	>20%	Consider conduction block or anomalous innervation.
CMAP or SNAP amplitude side-to-side difference	>50%	Consider axonal injury.

[a]Summation of the median and ulnar sensory antidromic conduction onset difference to the ring finger at 14 cm (ringdiff) + the median and radial sensory antidromic conduction difference to the thumb at 10 cm (thumbdiff) + the median and ulnar orthodromic conduction difference across the wrist with palmar stimulation at 8 cm (palmdiff).

CHAPTER 26

Reimbursement

Jay M. Weiss

This chapter is written to provide guidelines for electrodiagnostic reimbursement issues. It is difficult to adequately cover all aspects of this topic in a few pages. Two terms must be defined when discussing reimbursement: *coding* and *billing*. There are books and journals that deal exclusively with these issues. Coding is the process of transforming diagnoses and procedures into numeric codes, while billing is the process of transmitting the correct diagnosis and procedure codes to the payer. It is important to note that proper documentation in the medical record is an essential part of coding and billing. Your medical notes and reports must support your selection of diagnostic and procedural codes.

The electrodiagnostic evaluation is a complex, time-consuming examination requiring real-time interpretation of data and continual reassessment and modification of which nerves and muscles are to be tested. Electrodiagnostic studies are individually designed by the EDX physician for each patient.[1] It also requires highly specialized computerized equipment and expert knowledge regarding the technology. As such, electrodiagnostic evaluation should be appropriately reimbursed for a test requiring this level of skill, training, knowledge, time, and equipment.

The electrodiagnostic consultation is an extension of the neurologic portion of the physical examination. It is essential for the electromyographer to perform a history and physical examination as part of the study. Sometimes all that is necessary is a brief pretest history and focused physical examination. According to the American Association of Neuromuscular and Electrodiagnostic Medicine (AANEM), a brief pretest history and focused physical examination is part of a standard electrodiagnostic (EDX) evaluation.[2] If this brief evaluation is not adequate, a more detailed evaluation is necessary. If such an examination is performed and documented, it is entirely appropriate to bill for the examination under the Medical Evaluation and Management Codes. These are the same codes used to describe office visits and consultations. Usually codes 99202 to 99205 (for initial office visits) or codes 99242 to 99244 (for consultations) would be used. It should be pointed out that Medicare no longer accepts codes 99242 to 99245 (consultation codes), and in such cases a consultation should be coded using the appropriate office visit code (generally 99202 to 99205).

Before we discuss billing, we must tackle the issue of coding. Most insurance companies and Medicare carriers require all listed procedures and diagnoses to be provided in the form of alphanumeric codes, because computers can more easily process these codes (rather than narrative descriptions). The importance of proper coding cannot be overstated. Insurance carriers will deny or reimburse electrodiagnostic procedures based on the diagnostic code used. Often there are several diagnosis codes that may fit a clinical picture. There are generalized codes for pain or numbness in a limb and more specific codes for peripheral entrapments or radiculopathies. In instances where there is neck pain and clinical evidence of radiculopathy, it is better to use the radiculopathy code than the neck pain code, because generic neck pain may or may not merit electrodiagnostic studies but radiculopathies most often will. You may choose to use more than one diagnostic code.

Where Do These Codes Originate?

The last few years have seen drastic changes in coding for electrodiagnosis. In most cases, an electromyography (EMG) study performed today would use few of the codes used just a few years ago for the same study. In this chapter, every effort has been made to use codes that are current as of the date of publication; however, the codes used can and do change over time. Therefore, it is incumbent upon the physician and other healthcare professionals to remain up to date on current acceptable coding and billing practices.

For *diagnosis* codes, there are many books and other references that list ICD-10 codes (International Classification of Diseases 10th Edition by the World Health Organization). Most hospitals also have experts on staff (professional coders) who are able to provide further education about how to properly use these codes. For *procedural* codes, there is a reference book titled the Current Procedural Terminology[3] (CPT) Manual that is published annually by the American Medical Association (AMA) and attempts to most accurately describe *procedures*. For the most commonly used electrodiagnostic codes, see Table 26.1. The AMA's CPT Manual frequently eliminates, revises, and/or creates new codes. As a practical matter, some insurance carriers or systems may not recognize all current CPT codes; some may use eliminated codes. For example, the New York State Workers' Compensation fee schedule continued to use the discontinued EMG/NCS (nerve conduction study) codes for many years, only recently adopting the changes made years ago. In specific instances, it may be necessary to discuss individual coding questions with the carrier to find their closest acceptable code.

TABLE 26.1 ▪ Current Procedural Terminology (CPT®) Codes in Electrodiagnostic Medicine[2]

95885	Needle electromyography, each extremity, with related paraspinal areas, when performed, done with nerve conduction, amplitude and latency/velocity study; limited
95886	Needle electromyography, each extremity, with related paraspinal areas, when performed, done with nerve conduction, amplitude and latency/velocity study; complete, five or more muscles studied, innervated by three or more nerves or four or more spinal levels
95887	Needle electromyography, non-extremity (cranial nerve supplied or axial) muscle(s) done with nerve conduction, amplitude and latency/velocity study
95860[a]	Needle electromyography; one extremity with or without related paraspinal areas
95861[a]	Needle electromyography; two extremities with or without related paraspinal areas
95863[a]	Needle electromyography; three extremities with or without related paraspinal areas
95864[a]	Needle electromyography; four extremities with or without related paraspinal areas
95867	Needle electromyography cranial nerve supplied muscle(s) unilateral
95868	Needle electromyography cranial nerve supplied muscle(s) bilateral
95869	Needle electromyography thoracic paraspinal muscles (excluding T1 or T12)
95870	Needle electromyography limited study of muscles in one extremity or non-limb (axial) muscles (unilateral or bilateral), other than thoracic paraspinal, cranial nerve supplied muscles, or sphincters.

Nerve Conduction Studies

95907	1–2 nerve conduction studies
95908	3–4 nerve conduction studies
95909	5–6 nerve conduction studies
95910	7–8 nerve conduction studies
95911	9–10 nerve conduction studies
95912	11–12 nerve conduction studies
95913	13 or more nerve conduction studies

[a]Use electromyography (EMG) codes (95860–95864 and 95867–95870) when no nerve conduction studies (95907–95913) are performed on that day. Use 95885, 95886, and 95887 for EMG services when nerve conduction studies (95907–95913) are performed in conjunction with EMG on the same day.

Using the Procedure Codes

According to the current rules, when billing for nerve studies, the clinician must count up the total number of nerve studies performed and translate that into a code. There are different nerve study codes that indicate the number of nerves examined; however, only one nerve study code can be billed without a multiplier. For example, if four nerve studies are performed, code 95908 must be used (three to four nerve studies), rather than code 95907 (one to two nerve studies) with a multiplier of 2. Therefore, only one code from 95907 to 95913 can be used, and this can only be used once a day.

Multiple stimulation sites on the same nerve are all part of one nerve study and should be counted only once. In other words, a median motor nerve study with electrodes over the abductor pollicis brevis and stimulations at the wrist, elbow, axilla, and Erb's point counts as *one nerve study*. F-waves are not counted separately and a motor nerve study with or without an F-wave is one study. H-reflexes are no longer billed as separate codes, but each H-reflex counts as one nerve study. Therefore, if a right and a left H-reflex are performed, these count as two nerve studies and should be added to the total number of motor and sensory nerve studies.

For example, median motor and sensory studies of both upper extremities and ulnar motor and sensory studies of both upper extremities would be a total of eight nerve studies. This is the same number (eight studies) whether F-waves are used or not. In another example, a right fibular nerve study with stimulation at the ankle and fibular head, along with a right tibial motor nerve study with stimulation at the ankle and popliteal fossa, counts as two nerve studies. If bilateral sural nerves are studied and bilateral H-reflexes are performed, this is a total of six nerve studies and would correctly be coded as 95909. The total number of nerve studies performed is then translated into a code.

EMG codes 95860, 95861, 95863, and 95864 can be used when EMG is performed and no nerve studies are performed on that day. When EMG and nerve studies are performed at the same time, code 95886 or 95885 is used. The code 95886 is for a complete study of an extremity. It is defined as follows:

> *Needle electromyography, each extremity, with related paraspinal areas, when performed, done with nerve conduction, amplitude and latency/velocity study; complete, five or more muscles studied, innervated by three or more nerves or four or more spinal levels.*

Code 95886 can be billed more than once. If a limited EMG of a limb is performed (fewer than five muscles), it is 95885. Codes 95885 and 95886 can be used more than once, depending on the number of limbs examined. Codes 95885 and 95886 can both be billed in the same patient if one limb had a complete study and another had a limited study. They cannot both be billed for the same extremity.

The code for nonlimb muscles such as cranial muscles is CPT code 95887. It is defined as follows:

> *Needle electromyography, non-extremity (cranial nerve supplied or axial) muscle(s) done with nerve conduction, amplitude and latency/velocity study.*

Most carriers require (or at the very least, encourage) electronic submission. In these instances, your diagnosis and procedure codes are the only information the carrier will receive from you. Some carriers may request additional documentation. In other instances, the carrier may not realize that a code (e.g., 95886) can be billed more than once, so they may reimburse only one study. A review of the explanation of benefits portion of the claim may show that a code was denied as "repeat study" or "previously billed." In instances such as these, it would be helpful to send your report along with a copy of the CPT page noting that the code is "per extremity." You may have to educate the carrier or the claims representative as to the definitions of codes.

While it is the physician's decision to determine his or her own fees for procedures, in many instances (including Medicare and managed care plans), a physician agrees to accept a predetermined fee schedule. In cases of workers' compensation and motor vehicle accidents, many states have fixed fee schedules. The practitioner should be aware of the current testing fees in use in their geographic area. In some cases (such as workers' compensation in certain states), discontinued codes may still be in use. In such cases, the current Medicare and commercial insurance codes may not be in use for those systems.

Who Can Perform Electrodiagnostic Testing?

The details of electrodiagnostic studies are discussed elsewhere in this book. In terms of reimbursement, it is important to note that a needle EMG test is a dynamic test that is individualized to the clinical circumstance. Each of the 50 states has its own licensing and scope of practice criteria. The authors of this text agree with the AANEM opinion that state laws and regulations should define needle EMG as the practice of medicine to assure that patients undergoing these evaluations receive appropriate quality care. The AANEM's position is that electrodiagnostic evaluations should be performed by a physician (specifically a neurologist or physiatrist) who has had special training in the diagnosis and treatment of neuromuscular diseases and in the application of particular neurophysiologic techniques to the study of these disorders.[4] During the EMG study, different muscles may or may not be examined depending on the results of the study to that point. The working diagnosis is continually modified and reexamined based on the findings. Therefore the examination may be altered to confirm or refute different diagnoses.

As opposed to needle EMG (which should be performed by the physician), a technician, with physician supervision, can perform NCSs. However, it is important to note that it is the physician who must dictate the design of the study (choice of nerves) to fit the clinical circumstances. The physician is ultimately responsible for the analysis of the study. The physician should be available to confirm or refute any abnormal or unexpected findings. Both the electromyographer and the technician should be aware of the numerous technical factors that can produce false results.

In general, the EMG data is not recorded and cannot be independently reviewed and separately interpreted as can, for instance, an MRI of the spine. In this way it is different from many other diagnostic tests. It is most similar to a physical examination, where the only recording of the data is by the physician's record of the encounter. Thus the validity of any electrodiagnostic study is totally dependent on the knowledge, experience, and integrity of the electromyographer reporting the data.

Overuse of Studies

An electrodiagnostic consultation can be an expensive battery of tests, and unfortunately there have been problems with overuse and inappropriate use of electrodiagnostic studies. The cost of these studies, along with instances of inappropriate use and overuse, make these studies likely to come under close scrutiny. Ultimately, this can lead to insurance denials or partial denials of payment for appropriate studies. Thus it is important to be sure that the electrodiagnostic study is appropriate for the clinical picture.

An *adequate* number of nerve studies and needle insertions ensure the greatest degree of accuracy without undue discomfort or inappropriate expense. EMG testing of the extremity should be sufficient to refute or confirm a diagnosis. In most instances EMG should include the most symptomatic muscle or muscles (generally the weakest). If a symptomatic extremity is normal on EMG, examination of the asymptomatic extremity is not likely to be needed.

Nerve studies should be performed to provide specific information. Generally one or two motor and sensory nerves (in three extremities) are adequate in ruling out a generalized peripheral neuropathy. Beyond that, specific nerves can be helpful in evaluating a peripheral entrapment versus a more proximal lesion. In instances where a diagnosis of root avulsion is being considered,

TABLE 26.2 ■ **Maximum Number of Nerve Studies in Majority of Cases (for Selected Common Conditions, Based on AANEM Guidelines)**

Indication	Motor Studies	Sensory Studies	H-Reflex
Carpal tunnel (unilateral)	3	4	N/A
Carpal tunnel (bilateral)	4	6	N/A
Radiculopathy	3	2	2
Mononeuropathy	3	3	2
Polyneuropathy/mononeuropathy multiplex	4	4	N/A

AANEM, American Association of Neuromuscular and Electrodiagnostic Medicine.

sensory nerve studies can be crucial. In all cases there should be reasons based on the clinical circumstances for the nerve studies performed.

Peer Review Process

If there are questions as to the appropriateness of electrodiagnostic studies, the AANEM recommends the use of a peer review process. A physician with training in electrodiagnostic medicine should perform the peer review process for electrodiagnostic studies. Such a physician is almost always either a neurologist or a physiatrist (physicians who have completed a residency in neurology or physical medicine and rehabilitation). It is most appropriate for this specialist to be an experienced electromyographer who would therefore use the same criteria employed in his or her clinical practice. The AANEM has guidelines that suggest the numbers of nerve studies that should be adequate in greater than 90% of studies for a particular diagnosis. Studies that exceed these numbers could trigger peer review or other scrutiny (Table 26.2).

While the actual electrodiagnostic study cannot be reviewed for purposes of confirming or refuting the findings, a review of electrodiagnostic reports can be helpful in some circumstances. A review can address whether there were indications for the testing, and it can also note instances where the study was poorly designed. This can include a study that was too limited to fit the clinical circumstances or inadequate in its muscle selection. A review can address whether the conclusions were or were not supported by the data.

Summary

It is not enough merely to be a good electromyographer. The appropriate documentation in the medical record along with the selection of the diagnosis and procedure codes is necessary for obtaining proper reimbursement. The procedures performed should fit the clinical circumstances and should be adequate without being excessive. The procedures and indications should be adequately documented. By satisfying these criteria, the likelihood of proper reimbursement is maximized.

References

1. AANEM Position Statement. Recommended policy for electrodiagnostic medicine. Updated November 2019. https://www.aanem.org/Advocacy/Position-Statements/Recommended-Policy-for-Electrodiagnostic-Medicine_.
2. AANEM Position Statement. Billing for same day evaluation and management in electrodiagnostic testing. Updated November 2018.
3. Current Procedural Terminology (CPT) 2020. American Medical Association, 2019.
4. AANEM Position Statement. Who is qualified to practice electrodiagnostic medicine? Updated May 2012 and reapproved November 2017. https://www.aanem.org/Advocacy/Position-Statements/Who-is-Qualified-to-Practice-Electrodiagnostic-Med

Action potential: An electrical potential that moves along an axon or muscle fiber membrane.

Action potential morphology: The visual (display screen) appearance of the electrical activity recorded from a nerve or muscle as a result of nerve stimulation—commonly called a waveform.

Amplitude: The maximal height of the action potential (can be measured baseline to peak or peak to trough) that is expressed in millivolts (mV) for motor studies or microvolts (μV) for sensory studies.

Antidromic: When the electrical impulse travels in the opposite direction of normal physiologic conduction (e.g., conduction of a motor nerve electrical impulse away from the muscle and toward the spine, or a sensory study recorded distal to the stimulus).

Axonotmesis: Injury to the axon of a nerve but not to the supporting connective tissue. Results in Wallerian degeneration distal to the axonal injury.

Compound muscle action potential (CMAP): Summation of action potentials of muscle fibers recorded over a muscle following stimulation of a motor nerve.

Conduction block: Failure of an action potential to propagate past an area of injury, generally due to focal demyelination.

Conduction velocity: A measure of the speed of the fastest fibers in an action potential. (It can also be referred to as a motor conduction velocity or a sensory conduction velocity.)

Electrodiagnostic studies: Includes many tests (e.g., nerve conduction studies [NCS] and electromyography [EMG]) and is a physiological assessment of the electrical functioning of nerves and/or muscles.

Fasciculation potential: Spontaneous electrical potential originating in the nerve. Represents the spontaneous involuntary discharge of a single motor unit.

Fibrillation potential (fib): Spontaneous potential found on needle EMG testing at rest. Biphasic, initially positive deflection, originating in the muscle fiber.

Frequency: Cycles per second (frequently abbreviated Hertz or Hz).

F-wave: A compound muscle action potential evoked from antidromically stimulated motor nerve fibers using a supramaximal electrical stimulus. It generally represents only a small percentage of fibers and therefore is much smaller than an M-wave.

H-reflex: A compound muscle action potential evoked through orthodromic stimulation of sensory fibers and orthodromic activation of motor fibers. This potential is evoked with a submaximal stimulation and disappears with supramaximal stimulation. It is found in normal adults only in the gastrocnemius–soleus and flexor carpi radialis muscles. The response is thought to be due to a mono- or oligosynaptic spinal reflex (Hoffmann reflex).

Insertional activity: The electrical activity generated as a result of disruption of the muscle membrane by a needle, which generally stops with the cessation of needle movement.

Latency: Time interval between the delivery of a stimulus and the onset of a response (the waveform's departure from baseline).

Late response: An evoked potential with a latency longer than an M-wave; includes H-reflexes and F-waves.

Miniature endplate potential: Potential produced spontaneously by the release of one quantum of acetylcholine from the presynaptic terminal.

Motor point: Area where the nerve enters the muscle (endplate zone).

Motor unit: Includes the anterior horn cell, as well as its axon, neuromuscular junction, and all the muscle fibers innervated by that axon.

Motor unit action potential (MUAP): A motor unit action potential is the electrical activity (recorded or observed) corresponding to the firing of one motor unit. This represents the summation of the electrical activity of the muscle fibers supplied by one axon.

M-wave: Muscle action potential evoked by stimulating a motor nerve.

Myokymic discharge: Motor unit action potentials that fire repetitively (often referred to as sounding like marching soldiers).

Myopathic recruitment: Early recruitment (an increased number) of motor unit action potentials for the strength of contraction. Frequently seen in myopathies (in which the motor unit amplitudes are typically decreased).

Myotonic discharge: High frequency discharges whose amplitude and frequency wax and wane (sometimes referred to as "dive bombers").

Nerve conduction studies (NCS): Assessment of nerve function via electrical stimulation.

Neurapraxia: A lesion where conduction block is present and the axon remains intact.

Neurotmesis: A complete injury of a nerve (e.g., a transection) involving the myelin, axon, and all of the supporting structures.

Orthodromic: When the electrical impulse travels in the same direction as normal physiologic conduction (e.g., when a motor nerve electrical impulse is transmitted toward the muscle and away from the spine or when a sensory nerve impulse is recorded proximal to the point of stimulation).

Positive sharp wave (PSW): Primarily monophasic spontaneous potential found on EMG at rest, initially positive deflection with a characteristic "V" formation. Originates in the muscle fiber.

Recruitment: The orderly addition of motor units with increasing voluntary muscle contraction.

Sensory nerve action potential (SNAP): Summation of action potentials recorded from the nerve following stimulation of a sensory nerve.

Stimulus: An electrical depolarization of a nerve initiating an action potential. A stimulus can be supramaximal or submaximal.

Submaximal stimulus: An electrical stimulus that results in the initiation of an action potential in some, but not all, of the nerve fibers. Increasing the intensity of a submaximal stimulus will change the appearance of the CMAP or SNAP.

Supramaximal stimulus: An electrical stimulus that results in the initiation of an action potential in all fibers of the targeted nerve. Increasing the intensity of a supramaximal stimulus will not change the appearance of the CMAP or SNAP.

Temporal dispersion: Long-duration, low-amplitude action potential due to extreme variations in the conduction velocities of individual nerve fibers contributing to the action potential.

Figures for Table 4.3 (Nerve Conduction Studies Setup)

When one stimulation site is given, it refers to the cathode location. The anode is generally proximal to the cathode. For late responses (F-wave and H-reflex), the cathode is proximal and the anode is distal.

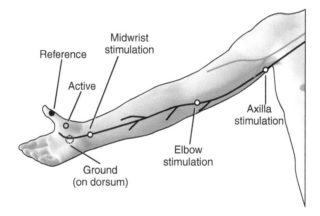

Fig. A1.1 Median nerve—motor.

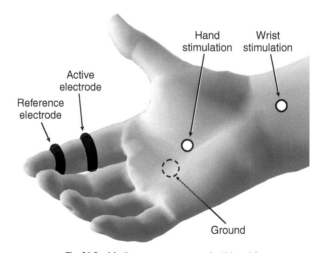

Fig. A1.2 Median nerve—sensory (antidromic).

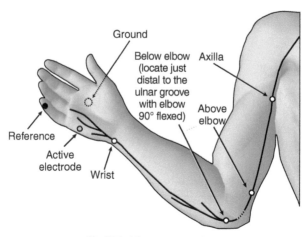

Fig. A1.3 Ulnar nerve — motor.

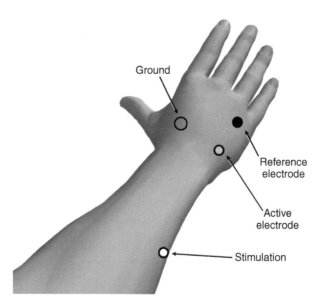

Fig. A1.4 Dorsal ulnar cutaneous nerve — sensory (orthodromic).

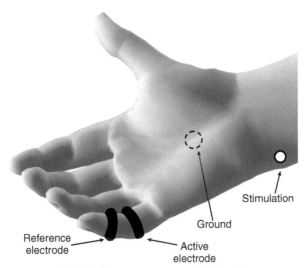

Fig. A1.5   Ulnar nerve — sensory (antidromic).

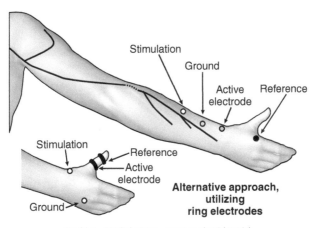

Fig. A1.6   Radial nerve — sensory (antidromic).

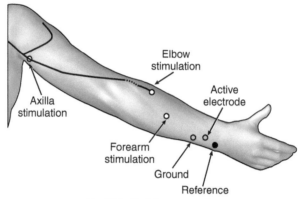

Fig. A1.7   Radial nerve—motor.

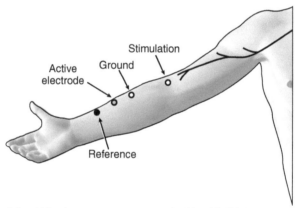

Fig. A1.8   Lateral antebrachial cutaneous nerve—sensory (antidromic). This is a sensory branch from the musculocutaneous nerve.

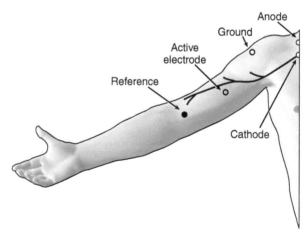

Fig. A1.9   Musculocutaneous nerve—motor.

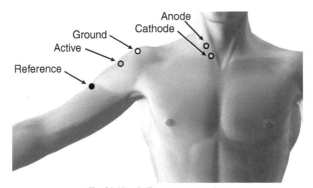

Fig. A1.10　Axillary nerve — motor.

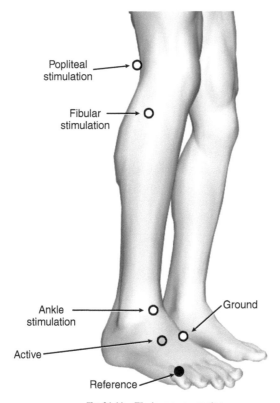

Fig. A1.11　Fibular nerve — motor.

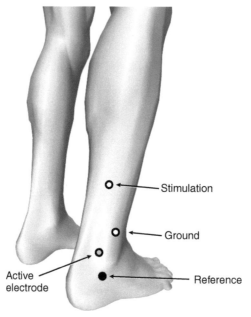

Stimulation

Ground

Active
electrode

Reference

Fig. A1.12   Sural nerve—sensory.

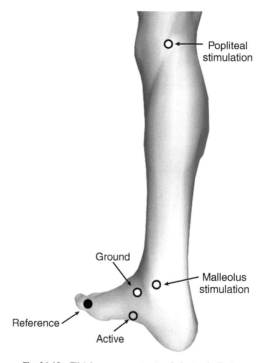

Popliteal
stimulation

Ground

Malleolus
stimulation

Reference

Active

Fig. A1.13   Tibial nerve—motor to abductor hallucis.

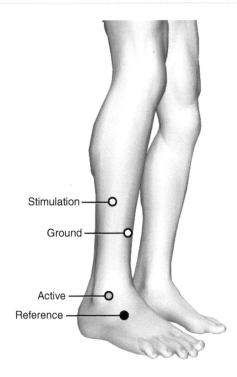

Stimulation —○

Ground —○

Active —○

Reference —●

Fig. A1.14 Superficial fibular nerve—sensory (antidromic).

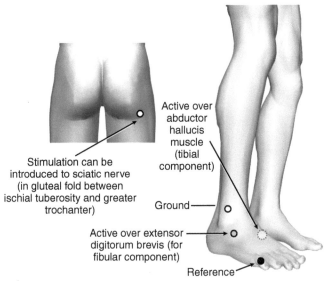

○ Active over abductor hallucis muscle (tibial component)

Stimulation can be introduced to sciatic nerve (in gluteal fold between ischial tuberosity and greater trochanter)

Ground —○

Active over extensor —○ digitorum brevis (for fibular component)

Reference —●

Fig. A1.15 Sciatic nerve—motor.

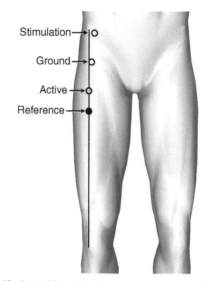

Fig. A1.16 Lateral femoral cutaneous nerve—sensory (antidromic).

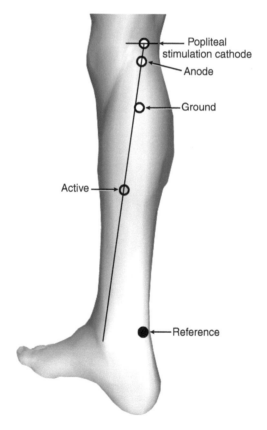

Fig. A1.17 H-reflex.

Figures for Table 5.4 (Common Muscles—Innervation, Location, and Needle Placement)

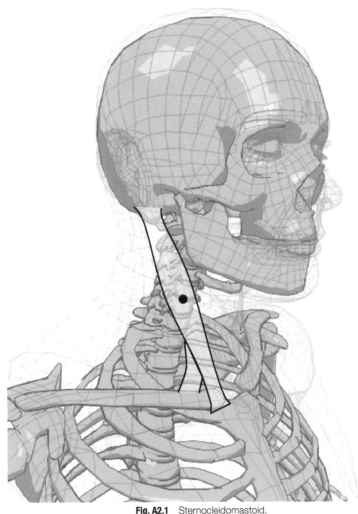

Fig. A2.1 Sternocleidomastoid.

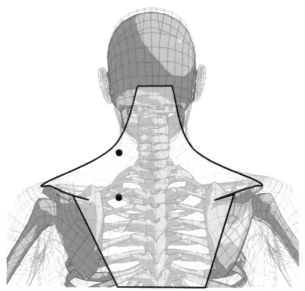

Fig. A2.2 Trapezius.

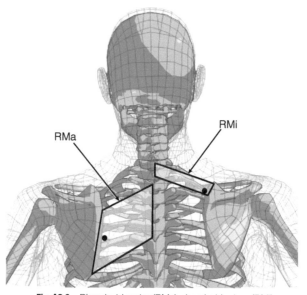

Fig. A2.3 Rhomboid major (RMa); rhomboid minor (RMi).

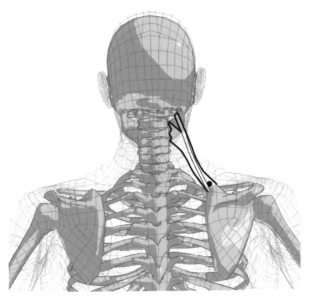

Fig. A2.4   Levator scapulae.

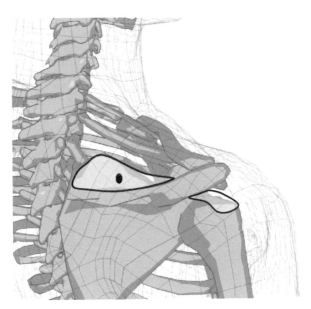

Fig. A2.5   Supraspinatus.

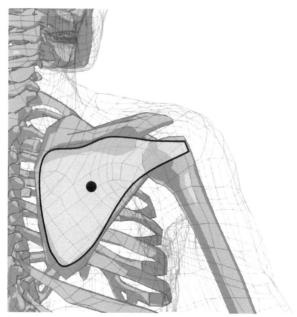

Fig. A2.6 Infraspinatus.

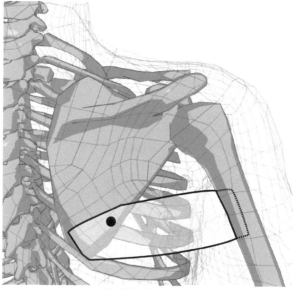

Fig. A2.7 Teres major.

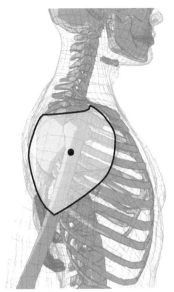

Fig. A2.8 Deltoid.

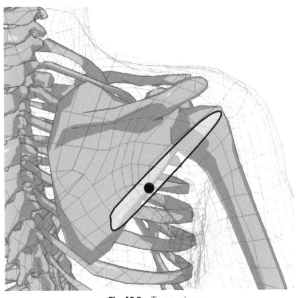

Fig. A2.9 Teres minor.

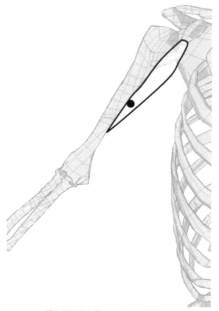

Fig. A2.10 Coracobrachialis.

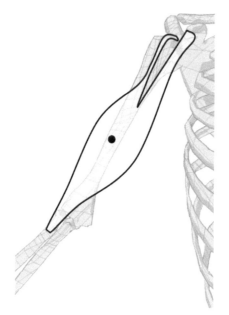

Fig. A2.11 Biceps brachii.

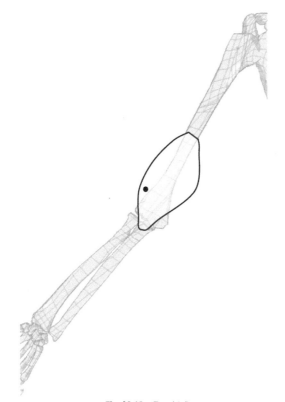

Fig. A2.12   Brachialis.

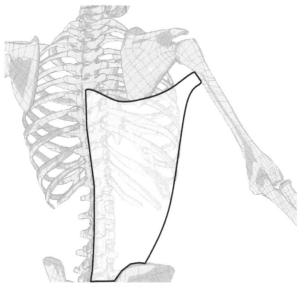

Fig. A2.13   Latissimus dorsi.

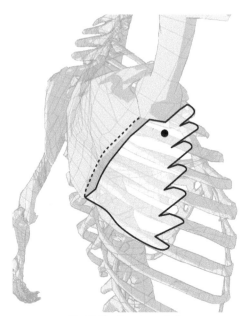

Fig. A2.14   Serratus anterior.

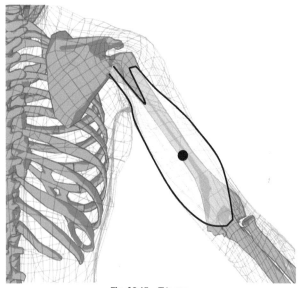

Fig. A2.15   Triceps.

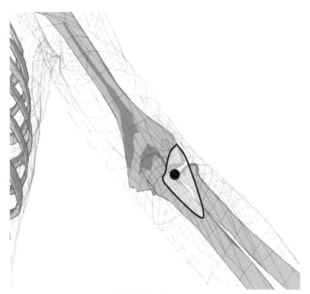

Fig. A2.16 Anconeus.

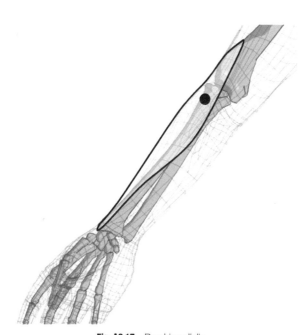

Fig. A2.17 Brachioradialis.

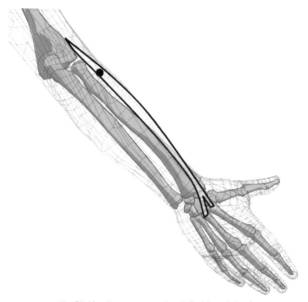

Fig. A2.18   Extensor carpi radialis (dorsal view).

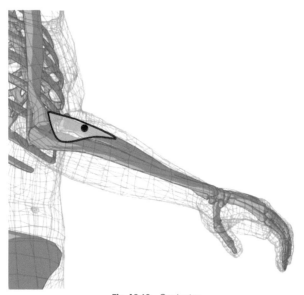

Fig. A2.19   Supinator.

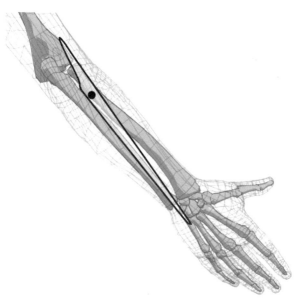

Fig. A2.20 Extensor carpi ulnaris (dorsal view).

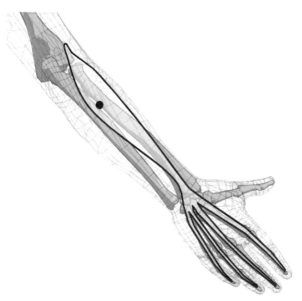

Fig. A2.21 Extensor digitorum (dorsal view).

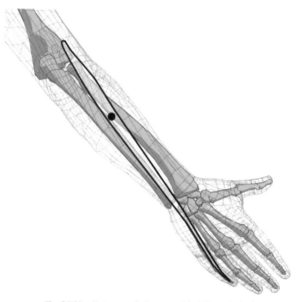

Fig. A2.22 Extensor digitorum minimi (dorsal view).

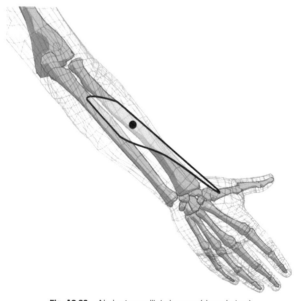

Fig. A2.23 Abductor pollicis longus (dorsal view).

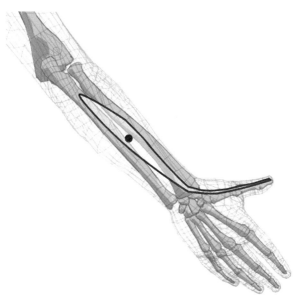

Fig. A2.24   Extensor pollicis longus (dorsal view).

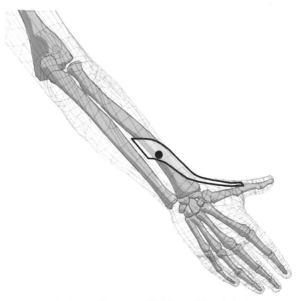

Fig. A2.25   Extensor pollicis brevis (dorsal view).

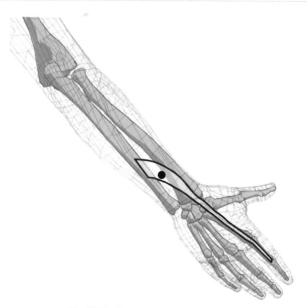

Fig. A2.26 Extensor indicis (dorsal view).

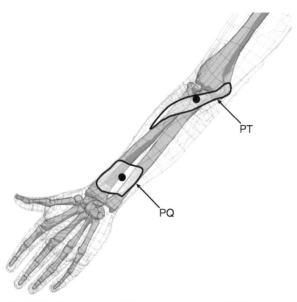

Fig. A2.27 Pronator teres (PT); pronator quadratus (PQ) (volar view).

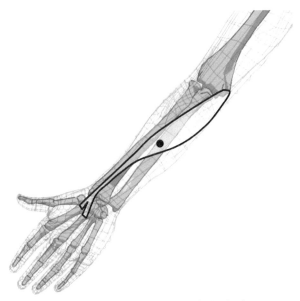

Fig. A2.28   Flexor carpi radialis (volar view).

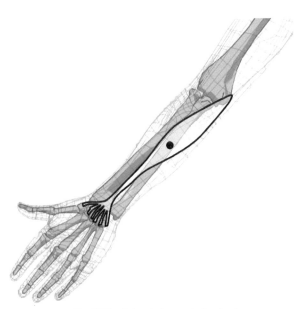

Fig. A2.29   Palmaris longus (volar view).

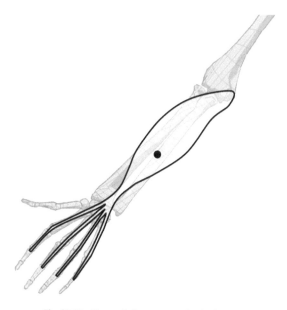

Fig. A2.30 Flexor digitorum superficialis (volar view).

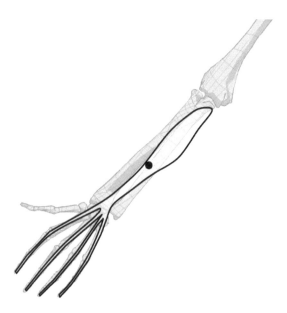

Fig. A2.31 Flexor digitorum profundus (volar view).

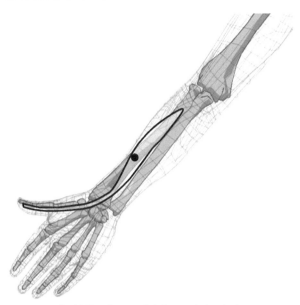

Fig. A2.32   Flexor pollicis longus (volar view).

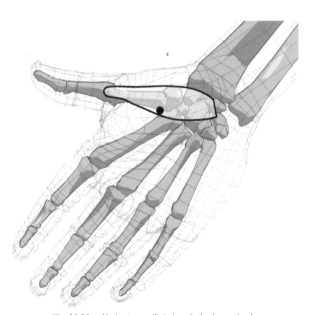

Fig. A2.33   Abductor pollicis brevis (palmar view).

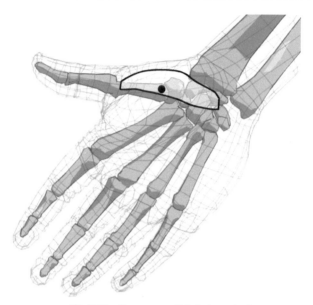

Fig. A2.34   Opponens pollicis (palmar view).

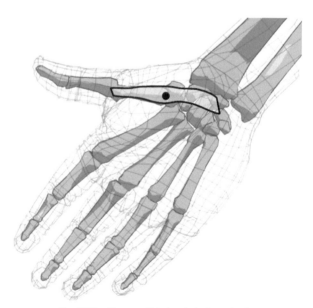

Fig. A2.35   Flexor pollicis brevis (palmar view).

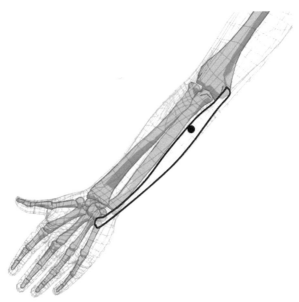

Fig. A2.36 Flexor carpi ulnaris (palmar view).

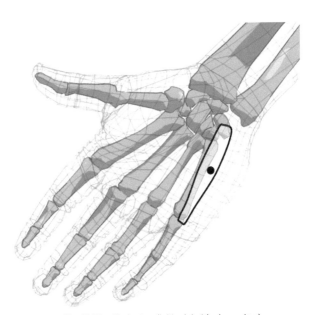

Fig. A2.37 Abductor digiti minimi (palmar view).

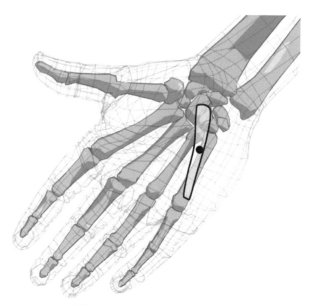

Fig. A2.38 Opponens digiti minimi (palmar view).

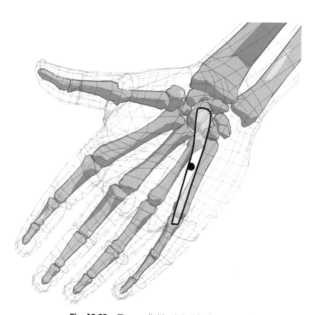

Fig. A2.39 Flexor digiti minimi (palmar view).

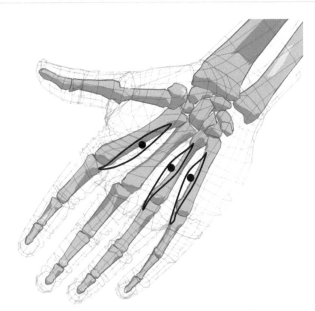

Fig. A2.40   Palmar interossei (palmar view).

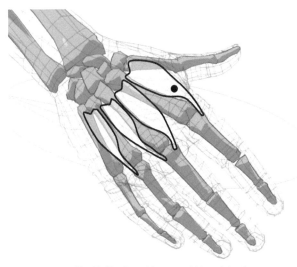

Fig. A2.41   Dorsal interossei (dorsal view).

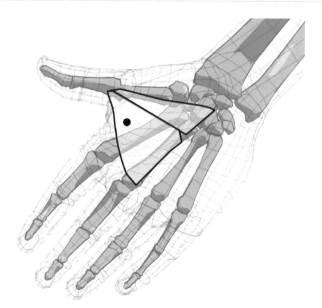

Fig. A2.42   Adductor pollicis (palmar view).

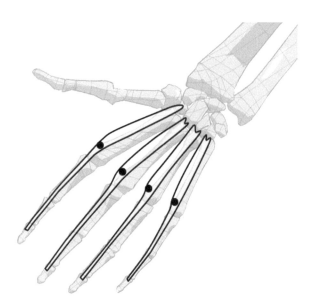

Fig. A2.43   Lumbricals (palmar view).

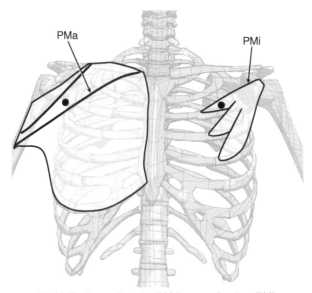

Fig. A2.44   Pectoralis major (PMa); pectoralis minor (PMi).

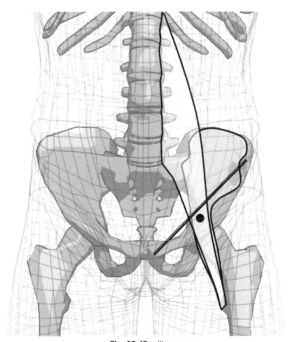

Fig. A2.45   Iliopsoas.

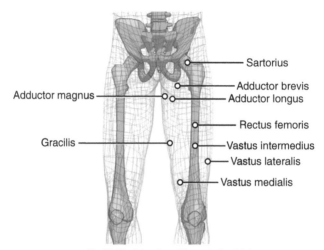

Sartorius

Adductor brevis

Adductor magnus

Adductor longus

Rectus femoris

Gracilis

Vastus intermedius

Vastus lateralis

Vastus medialis

Fig. A2.46   Muscles of the anterior thigh.

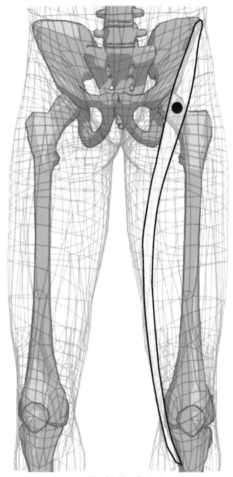

Fig. A2.47   Sartorius.

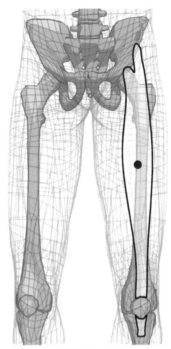

Fig. A2.48   Rectus femoris.

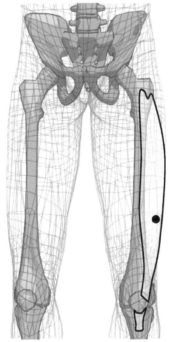

Fig. A2.49   Vastus lateralis.

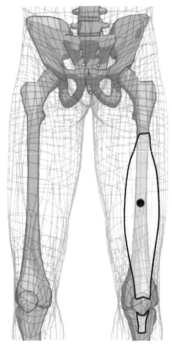

Fig. A2.50 Vastus intermedius.

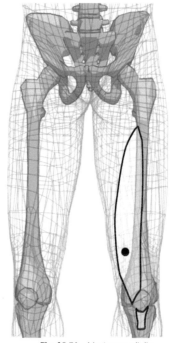

Fig. A2.51 Vastus medialis.

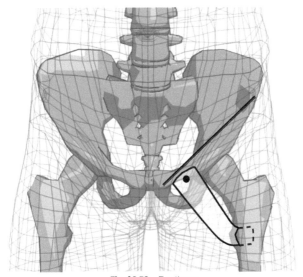

Fig. A2.52 Pectineus.

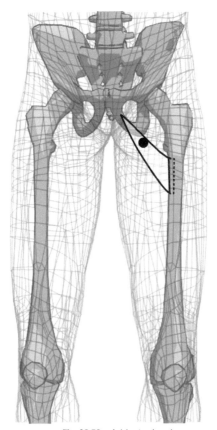

Fig. A2.53 Adductor brevis.

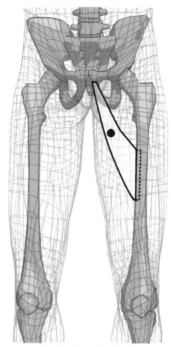

Fig. A2.54 Adductor longus.

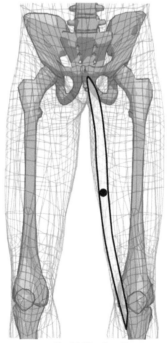

Fig. A2.55 Gracilis.

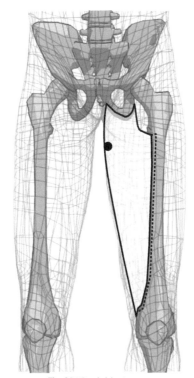

Fig. A2.56   Adductor magnus.

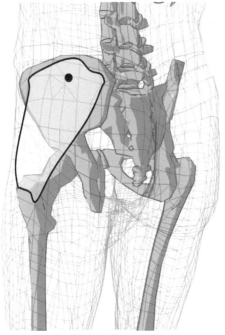

Fig. A2.57   Gluteus medius.

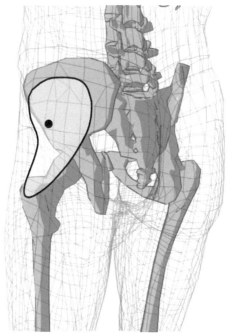

Fig. A2.58 Gluteus minimus.

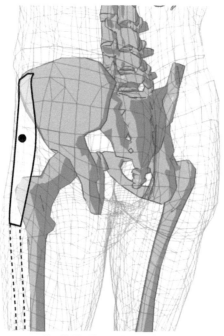

Fig. A2.59 Tensor fasciae latae.

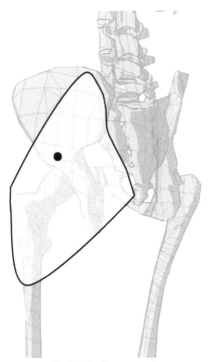

Fig. A2.60 Gluteus maximus.

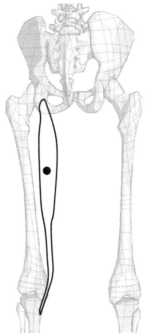

Fig. A2.61 Semitendinosus.

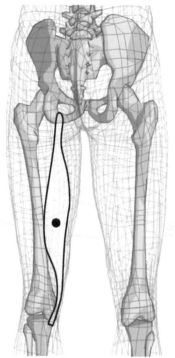

Fig. A2.62   Semimembranosus.

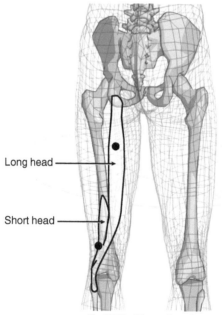

Long head

Short head

Fig. A2.63   Biceps femoris.

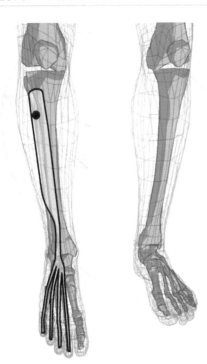

Fig. A2.64 Extensor digitorum longus.

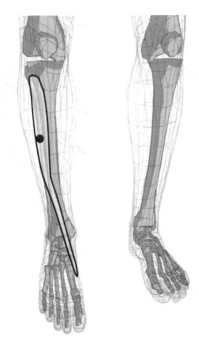

Fig. A2.65 Tibialis anterior.

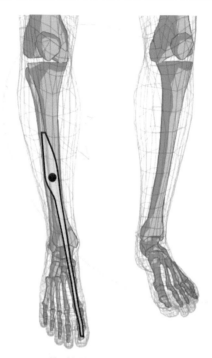

Fig. A2.66 Extensor hallucis longus.

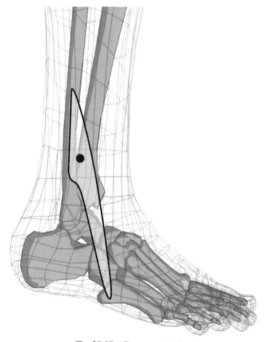

Fig. A2.67 Peroneus tertius.

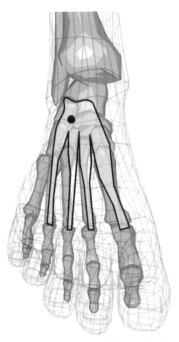

Fig. A2.68 Extensor digitorum brevis.

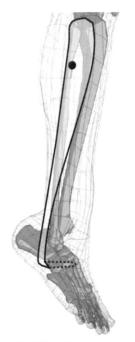

Fig. A2.69 Peroneus longus.

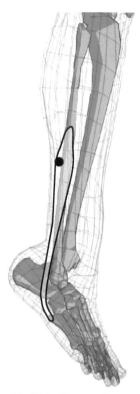

Fig. A2.70   Peroneus brevis.

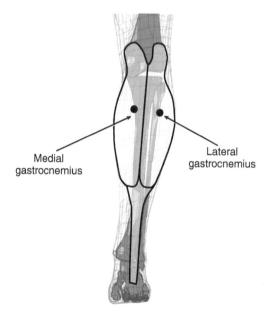

Medial
gastrocnemius

Lateral
gastrocnemius

Fig. A2.71   Medial and lateral gastrocnemius.

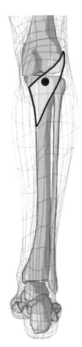

Fig. A2.72   Popliteus.

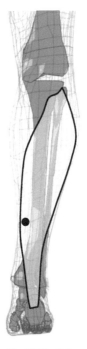

Fig. A2.73   Soleus.

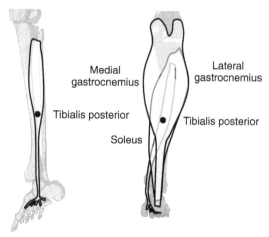

Fig. A2.74 Muscles of the calf.

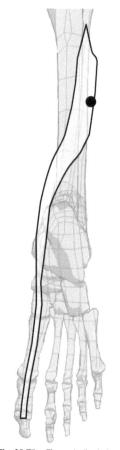

Fig. A2.75 Flexor hallucis longus.

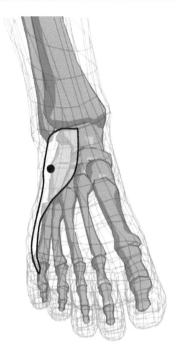

Fig. A2.76 Abductor digiti minimi.

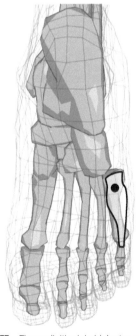

Fig. A2.77 Flexor digiti minimi (plantar surface).

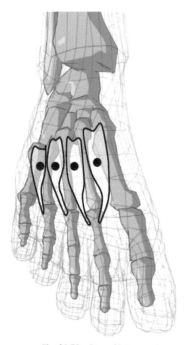

Fig. A2.78 Dorsal interossei.

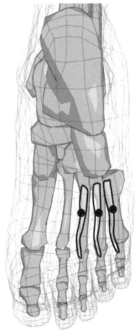

Fig. A2.79 Plantar interossei (plantar surface).

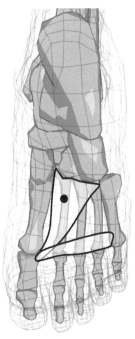

Fig. A2.80   Adductor hallucis (plantar surface).

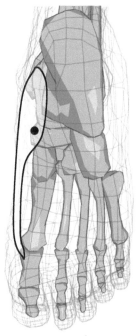

Fig. A2.81   Abductor hallucis (plantar surface).

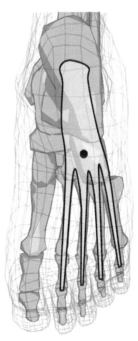

Fig. A2.82   Flexor digitorum brevis (plantar surface).

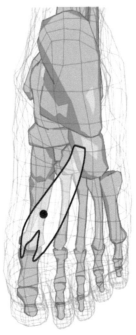

Fig. A2.83   Flexor hallucis brevis (plantar surface).

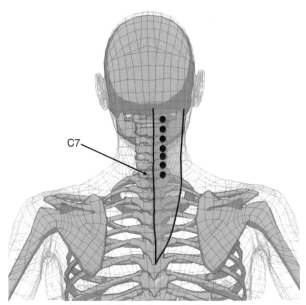

Fig. A2.84 Cervical paraspinal muscles.

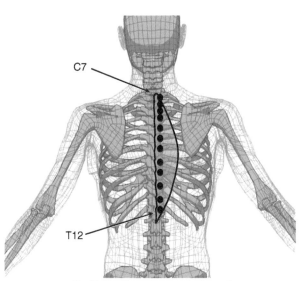

Fig. A2.85 Thoracic paraspinal muscles.

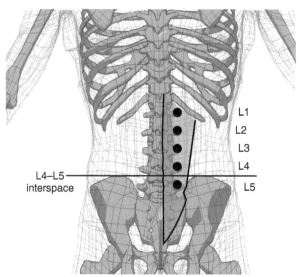

Fig. A2.86   Lumbosacral paraspinal muscles.

Summary of Electrodiagnostic Findings in Specific Clinical Conditions

Disorder	Sensory NCS	Motor NCS	Needle Study	Special Tests	Special Considerations
Carpal tunnel syndrome, sensory only	Slowing of the median nerve segment across the wrist but not midpalm to digit 2 with normal ulnar velocities OR decreased median amplitude but not ulnar.	Normal	Normal	Combined sensory index or bactrian sign may be positive in mild sensory CTS and help identify the disorder.	
Carpal tunnel syndrome, sensorimotor	Slowing of the median nerve segment across the wrist but not midpalm to digit 2 with normal ulnar velocities OR decreased median amplitude but not ulnar.	Prolonged distal median latency with normal ulnar distal motor latency, significant side-to-side amplitude decrease suggest a neurapraxic or axonotmetic lesion.	Normal	None	A distal conduction block is possible. If the amplitudes are low compared to the ulnar amplitudes but no denervation is present, consider a distal conduction block of the median nerve at the wrist. CSI (or other comparative study such as "bactrian" may be the earliest electrodiagnostic (EDX) abnormality.
Carpal tunnel syndrome, severe	Slowing of the median nerve segment across the wrist but not midpalm to digit 2 with normal ulnar velocities OR decreased median amplitude but not ulnar.	Prolonged distal median latency with normal ulnar distal motor latency.	Denervation* in the APB muscle but NOT in ulnarly innervated hand muscles (also C8–T1) and NOT in proximal median innervated muscles (pronation teres).	None	If ulnar muscles have denervation, consider a C8–T1 radiculopathy. If the pronator teres is involved, consider a proximal median nerve lesion.

Disorder	Sensory NCS	Motor NCS	Needle Study	Special Tests	Special Considerations
Peripheral neuropathy— see Fig. 16.1					
Ulnar neuropathy at the elbow (cubital tunnel syndrome)	May have decreased ulnar sensory amplitudes. The dorsal ulnar cutaneous nerve should be affected as well.	Slowing or amplitude drop of the ulnar motor nerve across the elbow but not elsewhere. "Inching" may be helpful.	Normal unless axonal damage is present. Then all ulnar muscles distal to the lesion will have denervation. However, the only ulnarly innervated muscles in the forearm are the FCU and the FDP to digits 4 and 5. The FCU and the FDP MAY be innervated proximal to the elbow.		If a conduction block (neurapraxia) is present, distal amplitudes will be low only when stimulating proximal to (across) the block.
Ulnar neuropathy at the wrist (Guyon's canal)	Decreased amplitude depending on the level of the plexopathies. Sensory distal latencies and conduction velocities should be normal. The medial antebrachial cutaneous nerve may be affected (low amplitude) with medial cord or lower trunk lesions. The lateral antebrachial cutaneous nerve may be affected in lateral cord or upper trunk lesions.	Prolonged distal ulnar latency with normal distal median motor latency. Consider pickup over the first dorsal interossei.	Normal unless axonal damage is present. Then all ulnar muscles in the hand will have denervation except the lumbricals to digits 4 and 5, which come off the FDP proximal to the wrist. The FDI may show more abnormalities than the ADM.	Consider pickup over the FDI muscle in addition to the ADM, as the FDI muscle is more likely to be involved.	

Disorder	Sensory NCS	Motor NCS	Needle Study	Special Tests	Special Considerations
Brachial plexopathy		May see slowing of conduction velocity across Erb's point, as well as decreased CMAP amplitude of the affected distal peripheral nerves.	Denervation in muscles distal to the level of injury (that receive innervation from that segment) with normal paraspinal muscles.	F-waves are not indicated as most lesions are incomplete and will have some fibers with normal conduction velocities. A small and localized slowing would be diluted by the long path of the F-wave. Furthermore, commonly performed F-waves (median and ulnar) are only carried by the lower trunk and medial cord and not the upper or middle trunk or lateral or posterior cord.	F-waves abnormalities are NOT diagnostic of a radiculopathy or a plexopathy, as (1) most muscles are innervated by at least two root levels and the unaffected nerve root will conduct normally. (2) Slowing anywhere along the pathway may lead to a prolonged F-wave latency (i.e., a median neuropathy such as carpal tunnel will lead to a prolonged F-wave if pickup is at the APB muscle). (3) F-waves test a very long segment of nerve. Slowing of a small proximal segment is usually washed out by the long segment. (4) F-waves are variable and nonspecific. Lesions at the trunk level may be distinguished from cord level lesions by the involvement of antagonist muscles at the trunk level.
Cervical radiculopathy	Normal sensory responses as the lesion is proximal to the dorsal root ganglion.	Usually normal. Most muscles are innervated by at least two nerve roots. In order to have a 50% side-to-side amplitude difference (which would be considered significant), more than 50% of the nerve would have to be affected.	Denervation in the cervical paraspinal muscles plus denervation in at least two muscles innervated by that root but different peripheral nerves constitutes a definitive diagnosis.	An H-reflex may be elicited from the FCR muscle stimulating the median nerve at the elbow. F-waves are not indicated as they are not sensitive or specific.	

Disorder	Sensory NCS	Motor NCS	Needle Study	Special Tests	Special Considerations
Tibial neuropathy at the ankle (tarsal tunnel syndrome)	Decreased amplitudes or slowing of medial and/or lateral plantar nerves with sparing of the calcaneal branch. These mixed nerve responses are usually very small and difficult to obtain and frequently require averaging. Compare affected to nonaffected side.	Prolonged distal latency of the tibial nerve at the ankle. If the medial branch is affected, pickup over the abductor hallucis may be affected. If the lateral plantar nerve is affected, pickup over the ADM may be affected.	Denervation may be seen in the foot muscles innervated by the tibial nerve if there is axonal damage.	It is important to test both medial and lateral plantar nerve fibers.	
Peroneal (fibular) neuropathy at the fibular head	Decrease amplitude of the superficial peroneal nerve may be noted if there is axonal injury. With a purely (or primarily) demyelinating lesion above the fibular head, sensory studies will be normal.	Distal conduction velocities may be normal if the slowing is proximal. Slowing of peroneal conduction across the fibular head may be noted. With a proximal conduction block, a drop in amplitude of the CMAP will be noted when stimulating above the lesion.	May see denervation of distal peroneal muscles if axonal injury is present.		It is important to test the short head of the biceps femoris. This muscle is innervated by the common peroneal nerve above the knee. Both superficial (peroneus longus and brevis) and deep peroneal muscles should be tested to assess if either or both branches are affected.

Disorder	Sensory NCS	Motor NCS	Needle Study	Special Tests	Special Considerations
Lumbosacral radiculopathy	Normal sensory responses as the lesion is proximal to the dorsal root ganglion.	Usually normal. Most muscles are innervated by at least two nerve roots. In order to have a 50% side-to-side amplitude difference (which would be considered significant), more than 50% of the nerve would have to be affected.	Denervation in the lumbar paraspinal muscles plus denervation in at least two muscles innervated by that root but different peripheral nerves constitutes a definitive diagnosis.	In S1 radiculopathy, the H-reflex on that side would be affected (prolonged latency or unobtainable). F-waves are not indicated as they are not sensitive or specific.	F-waves abnormalities are NOT diagnostic of a radiculopathy, as (1) Most muscles are innervated by at least two root levels and the unaffected nerve root will conduct normally. (2) Slowing anywhere along the pathway may lead to a prolonged F-wave (i.e., a sciatic neuropathy). (3) F-waves test a very long segment of nerve. Slowing of a small proximal segment is usually washed out by the long segment. (4) F-waves are variable and nonspecific.
Myopathy	Normal as only muscles (not sensory fibers) are affected.	Usually normal as pickup is on a distal (nonaffected) muscle. Distal latencies and conduction velocities will be normal.	Denervation may be noted in proximal muscles along with early recruitment of short duration, polyphasic, small amplitude motor units.		Needle testing may be normal in steroid myopathy as it involves type 2 fibers. Needle EMG assesses type 1 fibers.
AIDP (Guillain–Barré syndrome) and variants	Slowing of nerve conduction velocities, conduction block and prolongation of distal latencies may be noted. Sural nerves may be spared.	Slowing of nerve conduction velocities, conduction block, temporal dispersion, and prolongation of distal latencies may be noted.	In the axonal form of Guillain–Barré, denervation may be noted.	Prolonged or absent F-waves are usually the earliest electrodiagnostic findings.	While most Guillain–Barré is a demyelinating neuropathy, an axonal form occurs as well. Here, there would be more denervation and less slowing of nerve conduction velocity. A variant CIDP also exists.

Disorder	Sensory NCS	Motor NCS	Needle Study	Special Tests	Special Considerations
Motor neuron disease	Normal as the anterior horn cell (motor units) are affected.	May have decreased amplitudes, especially later in the disease when atrophy is present. Distal motor latencies and conduction velocities should be relatively normal, unless the fastest fibers are affected.	Denervation or fasciculation potentials in muscles innervated by at least three of the following areas: bulbar, cervical, thoracic, and lumbar. Motor units will have increased firing frequency (>10 Hz). In later stages of the disease, motor units may have longer duration, polyphasicity, and large amplitude. Acute and chronic changes may be noted.		It is important to sample muscles from multiple levels, proximal and distal.
Neuromuscular junction disorder MG, myasthenic syndrome, botulism	Normal, as there is no neuromuscular junction in a sensory nerve.	May see decreased amplitudes in Lambert–Eaton myasthenic syndrome.	In botulism, may see denervation. Instability of motor units (change in configuration) may be noted.	Repetitive nerve stimulation. A decrement in amplitude of the more than 10% from the first to the fifth waveform is seen. Note that since proximal muscles are affected more than distal muscles, this finding is usually seen more in proximal muscles. It is important to test at rest, after exercise (dramatic post exercise facilitation may be seen with Lambert–Eaton myasthenic syndrome) and then with recovery (postactivation exhaustion).	Since it is difficult to hold a stimulator in the exact same place with the same pressure, use a bar electrode as the stimulator. The patient should be off Mestinon for at least 24 hours. Make sure the limb is warm and make sure to test proximal and distal muscles.

Disorder	Sensory NCS	Motor NCS	Needle Study	Special Tests	Special Considerations
Sciatic neuropathy	Low amplitude of the sural nerve may be present. The sural nerve receives fibers from both the tibial and the peroneal nerve. The superficial peroneal nerve may also be affected. Distal latencies/ velocities should be normal if most of the nerve is preserved as lesion is proximal to stimulation.	Decreased amplitude of the tibial and peroneal nerves may be present. Distal latencies and conduction velocities should be normal.	Denervation in muscles innervated by the sciatic nerve distal to the lesion, as well as both the tibial and peroneal nerves.		
Radial neuropathy at the spiral groove	Decreased radial sensory amplitude.	If an axonal neuropathy is present, may see decreased amplitude of the radial motor CMAP. Slowing of conduction velocity may be seen across the lesion. With conduction block, there will be a drop in amplitude with stimulation proximal to the lesion.	May see denervation in all muscles except the triceps if there is an axonal lesion.		
Lateral femoral cutaneous neuropathy (meralgia paresthetica)	Increased latency and/ or decreased amplitude of the SSEP of the lateral femoral cutaneous nerve.	Normal, as this is a pure sensory nerve.	Normal, as this is a pure sensory nerve.	Somatosensory evoked potential is a better test than sensory nerve studies for this disorder. A side-to-side difference in latency or decreased amplitude may be seen. Since the involved pathway is long and involves more than just the lateral femoral cutaneous nerve, the test is sensitive but not specific.	

Disorder	Sensory NCS	Motor NCS	Needle Study	Special Tests	Special Considerations
Anterior interosseous neuropathy	Normal, as this is a motor nerve.	Normal if pickup is over the APB muscle, as it is not affected.	Denervation may be seen in the pronator quadratus, FDP (to digits 2 and 3) and flexor pollicis longus.	Motor studies of the median nerve can be performed with a needle in the pronator quadratus as the pickup electrode. Latency can be assessed in this manner, but amplitude is of limited usefulness.	
Supinator syndrome	Normal as the superficial radial nerve usually branches proximal to the supinator muscle.	If an axonal neuropathy is present, may see decreased amplitude of the radial motor CMAP. Slowing of conduction velocity may be seen across the lesion. With conduction block, there will be a drop in amplitude with stimulation above the lesion.	May see denervation in radial muscles distal to the supinator (the supinator muscle is spared as innervation is proximal to the muscle) if there is an axonal lesion.		
Femoral neuropathy	Decreased amplitude of the saphenous nerve.	May see decreased amplitude of the femoral CMAP with pickup over the quadriceps muscle. May see slowing of conduction velocity and conduction block across the lesion.	In an axonal lesion, may see denervation in all muscles innervated by the femoral nerve distal to the lesion. Needle EMG likely to be more helpful than nerve studies in femoral neuropathy.		

Disorder	Sensory NCS	Motor NCS	Needle Study	Special Tests	Special Considerations
Thoracic radiculopathy	Normal	Normal distal latency and conduction velocity in the extremities.	May see denervation in the thoracic paraspinal muscles at the level of the radiculopathy. Corresponding intercostal muscles may be affected as well.		
Spinal stenosis	Normally the dorsal root ganglia is usually spared.	Usually normal	Bilateral, multilevel root denervation may be noted, especially in the paraspinal muscles.	H-reflex may be prolonged or absent bilaterally if the S1 nerve root is affected.	
Critical illness neuropathy	Unobtainable motor responses or decreased sensory responses with near normal distal latency and conduction velocity.	Unobtainable motor responses or low amplitude motor responses with near normal distal latency and conduction velocity.	Denervation may be noted in distal muscles. This is an axonal neuropathy.		
Critical illness myopathy	Normal as only muscles (not sensory fibers) are affected.	Usually normal as pickup is on a distal (nonaffected) muscle.	Denervation may be noted in proximal muscles with early recruitment of short duration, polyphasic, small amplitude motor units.	Nerve conduction study of the phrenic nerve and needle study of the diaphragm may be indicated in patients who have difficulty weaning from the ventilator.	

*Denervation refers to abnormal spontaneous potentials (positive sharp waves and fibrillation potentials at rest) in the acute phase, and long duration, polyphasic motor units, or large motor units (consistent with denervation/ reinnervation) in the chronic phase.

ADM, Abductor digiti minimi; AIDP, acute inflammatory demyelinating polyneuropathy; APB, abductor pollicis brevis; CIDP, chronic inflammatory demyelinating polyneuropathy; CMAP, compound muscle action potentials; CSI, combined sensory index; CTS, carpal tunnel system; EMG, electromyography; FCR, flexor carpi radialis; FCU, flexor carpi ulnaris; FDI, first dorsal interosseous; FDP, flexor digitorum profundus; MG, myasthenia gravis; NCS, nerve conduction study; SSEP, somatosensory evoked potential.

Page numbers followed by "f" indicate figures, "t" indicate tables, and "b" indicate boxes.